Praise for *If You Wo...*

In this book, Joe Nowinski once again proves his ability to integrate the science and experience of Alcoholics Anonymous and to explain both in clear, unpretentious language.

—*Keith Humphreys, Professor of Psychiatry, Stanford University*

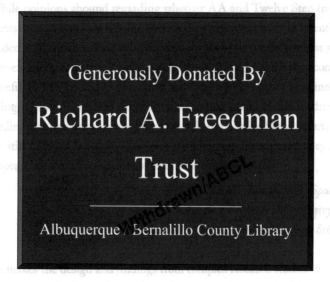

right amount of detail. The book thus represents a valuable new resource for anyone interested in a comprehensive summary of what we know about AA in terms of its effectiveness, its mechanisms of action, and its role in the existing arsenal of tools to support recovery.

—*Lee Kaskutas, Senior Scientist, Alcohol Research Group, Public Health Institute*

If You Work It,
It Works!

If You Work It, It Works!

THE SCIENCE BEHIND
12 STEP RECOVERY

JOSEPH NOWINSKI, PhD

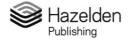

Hazelden Publishing

Hazelden Publishing
Center City, Minnesota 55012
hazelden.org/bookstore

ISBN: 978-1-61649-571-8; ebook 978-1-61649-574-9

Library of Congress Cataloging-in-Publication Data is on file
with the Library of Congress.

Editor's notes
The names, details, and circumstances may have been changed to protect the
privacy of those mentioned in this publication.

This publication is not intended as a substitute for the advice of health care
professionals.

Alcoholics Anonymous, AA, and the Big Book are registered trademarks of
Alcoholics Anonymous World Services, Inc.

19 18 17 16 15   1 2 3 4 5 6

Developmental editor: Sid Farrar
Production editor: Mindy Keskinen
Cover design by Theresa Gedig
Interior design by Terri Kinne
Typesetting by Bookmobile Design & Digital Publisher Services

Also by Joseph Nowinski

The Family Recovery Program
The Twelve Step Facilitation Handbook
The Twelve Step Facilitation Outpatient Program
Twelve Step Facilitation for the Dually Diagnosed Client

with Robert Doyle, MD
Almost Alcoholic: Is My or My Loved One's Drinking a Problem?

◆

For my parents
Joseph and Helen Nowinski
who showed me how to walk the walk . . .
and that has made all the difference.

Contents

Acknowledgments

I would like to acknowledge my editor, Sid Farrar of Hazelden Publishing, for his support for this as well as a previous book. Thanks, Sid, for being an excellent sounding board for ideas as well as a steadfast advocate for this book.

Prologue

As little as two decades ago, rigorous scientific research on the Alcoholics Anonymous (AA) Twelve Step program of recovery was all but nonexistent. It was so lacking, in fact, that a panel of experts convened by the Institute of Medicine of the National Academies (IOM) published this conclusion in 1989:

> Alcoholics Anonymous, one of the most widely used
> approaches to recovery in the United States, remains
> one of the least rigorously evaluated.

The IOM report went on to call for well-designed research studies aimed at evaluating the AA program. That is when fate crossed my path. Having received some training in the Twelve Step model of recovery, I had developed an adolescent treatment program rooted in that model and subsequently wrote a book about the experience. I was then invited to develop a parallel program for adults that would be used in a major national treatment outcome study. That study and its results will be included in the research we'll review here.

Suffice it to say that since the IOM report and the first published results of that national study, research on the AA program has proliferated, to the point where it is no longer true that AA is the least rigorously studied (or objectively evaluated) approach to recovery in the United States. However, to date much of the hard evidence regarding AA has been reported solely in academic journals, where it remains largely inaccessible to the general public. This book remedies that situation, shedding light on AA for all to see how it works. With that in mind, let's begin our tour of the science of Twelve Step recovery.

◆

Introduction

Problem or Solution?

It is hard to find someone who does not have an opinion about Alcoholics Anonymous—from those who say it has been their salvation to those who dismiss it as a harmful cult. Many people remain either skeptical or downright critical of AA. I know this from reading books and articles the critics have penned, and also from the responses I sometimes get to the blogs I post on sites such as The Huffington Post and Psychology Today.

I've come to divide these critics into two broad categories: those who claim that their criticism of the Twelve Step model is based on "scientific" evidence; and those whose criticism is merely their opinion—sometimes based on disappointing personal experiences. Here is an example, written in response to a blog I posted about how some college students drink heavily before going to a party (*frontloading*). Under the subject heading "Do you ever 'frontload'?" the commenter bitingly added,

> Then maybe you're an alcoholic. Another item to add to the alcoholism self-assessment checklist. You might have a "problem" so go to AA.
>
> Well, seriously we don't need more reasons to send people to AA, which is an unproven treatment and often just makes the problem worse (by requiring that the attendee admit "powerlessness" to their "cravings" among other things).

1

Frontloading is often just a way to save money, like the above commenter says, or to arrive at the party in a better mood, which is a perfectly good reason to drink. The real problem is chronic excessive drinking (front, back, or mid-loaded), which is normally a sign of an underlying psychological issue. In most cases it's just a phase that young people go through and does not lead to "alcoholism."

In the blog I had never mentioned AA, nor did I suggest that these students were destined to become alcoholics. Rather, I was writing about the increased risks associated with frontloading, such as fights, vandalism, and sexual assault. That did not deter this commentator, however, from gratuitously asserting that AA is an "unproven treatment" that "often just makes the problem worse."

Here is another typical criticism:

I would like to start by saying that I have attended a lot of 12 step meetings; in fact, the more 12 step meetings that I attended the worse my drinking became. I finally realized that AA was doing me a lot of harm when I had to check into medical detox so as not to die of the DTs [delirium tremens]. It was at this point that I left AA and started getting better.

Again, the idea proposed here is that AA and the Twelve Step program is actually harmful. Over the past several years I've read many such comments—some of them very biting, even bitter. I've often wondered exactly what kind of meetings these people attended, what their expectations were, and how sincere they were about wanting to quit drinking in the first place.

Then there are those—some of them credentialed professionals—who claim that AA does not help based on supposed "scientific" evidence. As an example, let me summarize a piece titled "AA Is Ruining the World."

> Here are four reasons AA is harmful and will hurt
> societies:
> - AA denies reality.
> - AA overemphasizes its own success.
> - AA rules out other, often more effective, approaches.
> - AA's underlying temperance message actually
>   creates alcoholism and addiction.

By this last criticism, the writer is arguing that in advocating for abstinence, AA actually promotes more drinking. Moreover, he asserts that he can prove this claim, though he does not cite that evidence. Nor have I been able to locate a body of objective research, or peer-reviewed treatment outcome studies, that this writer was associated with.

Here is another criticism of the Twelve Step program, this also from a professional—no less than a psychiatrist who was in charge of a major substance abuse treatment program:

> *AA has the worst success rate in all of medicine.*

And here is one more typical critique of AA:

> How much of the following do you recognize from AA?
> - treachery
> - disempowerment
> - infantilization
> - intimidation
> - stigmatization

The official response of the Alcoholics Anonymous central office to a steady stream of criticism like the above about its Twelve Step program of recovery can be summarized in one word: *silence*. That is because AA, by tradition, identifies itself as a "program of attraction"—if you work the Twelve Step program sincerely, AA believes it will work; conversely, if you don't like it, then by all means, try something else. (The Eleventh of the Twelve AA Traditions states, "Our public relations policy is based on attraction rather than promotion; we need always maintain personal anonymity at the level of press, radio, and films.") AA has never asserted that it works for everyone, only that "If you work it, it works."

Anonymity lies at the core of AA for two reasons. First, it serves to protect members who may worry that being publicly identified as an AA member could harm them in some way. This concern is legitimate, even though the stigma of alcoholism has declined among the general public in the recent past. Privately these individuals may indeed think of themselves as an "AA member" yet they are loath to be identified publicly that way.

The other reason that personal anonymity has remained so central to AA is that it impedes personal ambition, a desire to stand out, to accrue power or influence, or even to gain financially through AA. The result is that AA has remained steadfastly decentralized—and consequently very adaptable, as it is a bottom-up as opposed to a top-down organization. At the same time those traditions mean that no one individual speaks for AA. Unlike a corporation, a government agency, a political party, or even an organized religion, AA has no spokesperson, no press secretary.

AA's stance in this regard may not matter much to those who have found recovery through AA. They may simply regard these critics as ignorant. Yet AA's policy of silence has given its critics license to freely criticize both what AA is and how effective it is. Say what you will about AA, and AA will not offer a rebuttal.

So what do we say to all those men and women who may be troubled right now about their drinking behavior and are considering their options? What would we say to those who have been told that they must quit drinking or risk dire consequences in one form or another? What would these people be likely to conclude if they read only stinging criticisms like the above, while AA itself offers no retort? Unless they're willing to ignore such claims and try it for themselves, they may indeed assume that AA is an outdated, ineffective program and that stories about it working are either lies or the propaganda of its brainwashed members. Unless these people find help elsewhere, they're very likely to continue abusing alcohol or other drugs, and for many, this will mean falling deeper into the dangerous spiral of addiction and probable death.

This book addresses critics and criticisms like the above. It directly focuses on this underlying question: is AA and its Twelve Step program a dated, unproven approach to recovery from alcoholism and other addictions—or, as some would call it, a cult—or does it represent a real solution for one of the most challenging biological, psychological, and social problems that has plagued society for centuries?

Project MATCH

In 1990 I was invited by a research team at Yale University to design a treatment program for individuals with the diagnoses of alcohol abuse and alcohol dependence. This intervention needed to be based on the AA Twelve Step model of recovery. I was told that it would be used in a clinical trial investigating the effectiveness of the Twelve Step model. I had no idea at the time, however, of the magnitude of the research venture I was stepping into.

This study, named Project MATCH, was to be the most ambitious psychotherapy study ever undertaken. It was to be national in scope, involving nine separate treatment locations and nearly 2,000 patient/subjects. All of the participants had been diagnosed with an alcohol use disorder. Half of them were to be men and women who were recruited through ads in their communities (the "outpatient" group); the other half were to be recruited as they completed treatment programs (the "aftercare" group). A veritable *Who's Who* of alcohol treatment researchers (I did not count myself among them) were enlisted to design and implement the project.

My Twelve Step-based intervention, which I called Twelve Step Facilitation (TSF), was to be one of three interventions studied. The others were cognitive behavioral therapy (CBT) and motivational enhancement therapy (MET). The object of this study, which spanned seven years, was to determine not just if the three treatments were effective, but also what kind of treatment was most effective for what kind of patient (hence the inclusion of the word MATCH in the title).

The three treatments were chosen in part because they represented three different perspectives on how to treat what are now called *alcohol use disorders*. All three will be described in more detail later, but in a nutshell CBT is based on the idea that teaching such individuals coping skills will help them the most, because drinking represents a dysfunctional means of coping, for example with stress.

The MET perspective is different. It is based on the notion that men and women can and will find their own solutions for an alcohol use disorder, *once they decide they had one*. Accordingly, MET attempts to intervene in ways that lead these individuals to make that decision; for example, by pointing out negative consequences associated with their drinking.

Both CBT and MET already had been studied fairly extensively by the time MATCH went into development. In contrast, at that time Twelve Step-based interventions like the one I was asked to create had not been the subject of any significant, rigorous research. Although AA itself was ubiquitous and the Twelve Steps were an integral part of many facilities' treatment plans—especially those using what had come to be called the Minnesota Model—an actual formal treatment protocol based on the Twelve Step model and rigorously delivered by therapists was lacking. Moreover, in the academic community AA and the Twelve Step approach was poorly understood at best, with many academic researchers inclined to think of it more as a cult or quasi-religion than a serious programmatic approach to recovery from addiction. They were highly skeptical that TSF would work at all; or, if it did work, that it would do so only for those with the most severe alcohol use disorders (those men and women who had "bottomed out"). Nevertheless, TSF received the same resources and support for implementation as the other two interventions. So that was the atmosphere under which the first formal treatment protocol based on the AA Twelve Step program was developed and Project MATCH was launched.

Shortly after Project MATCH started, I was asked to be a contributor to a conference to be held at the Center on Alcoholism, Substance Abuse, and Addictions (CASAA) at the University of New Mexico. The impetus for this conference was the very same Institute of Medicine report asserting that AA and its Twelve Steps deserved more objective study than it had received.

The conference title was Research on Alcoholics Anonymous: Opportunities and Alternatives.

In an introduction to this conference, Barbara McCrady of Rutgers University and William R. Miller of the University of New Mexico wrote: "Although traditional controlled trials have not yet yielded evidence for the efficacy of AA, there are reasons to believe that something important is happening within AA, which needs to be better understood."

With these words in mind, the clinical and academic research communities alike were left to await the results of Project MATCH.

In 1997, seven years after work on it began, the Project MATCH Research Group published its first results: data on how effective the three treatments were for patients one year following treatment. The report stated that all three treatments were effective in reducing drinking and increasing abstinence at three months, six months, nine months, and twelve months following treatment. This in itself came as a surprise in many quarters, as it was once a common belief among health and mental health professionals that addicts and alcoholics were more or less doomed to relapse. MATCH demonstrated that this was not the case. One year after completing treatment, those in the outpatient arm of MATCH were sober slightly more than 80 percent of the time; meanwhile, those in the aftercare arm were sober 90 percent of the time. Contrary to some predictions, TSF was found to be equally effective for individuals who had been diagnosed as alcohol abusers (as opposed to full-fledged alcoholics). In other words, the Twelve Step model seemed not to be limited in its effectiveness to those who had bottomed out. Perhaps most surprising, however, was the finding that the Twelve Step approach, as embodied in TSF, held a slight *advantage* over both CBT and MET.

These findings were so unexpected that some long-standing critics of AA and its Twelve Step program went so far as to question whether the MATCH data were somehow falsified. Of course, nothing could be farther from the truth. The reality, rather, was what some skeptics simply could not abide: the idea that the Twelve Step approach works.

It is important to note that while Project MATCH focused exclusively on alcohol use disorders, in the intervening years all three of its treatments have been adapted for use with individuals whose issue is "polysubstance" use, meaning alcohol and other drugs. They have been adapted in this way to satisfy a clinical reality: that while some men and women still have only an alcohol problem, a great many are experiencing problems relating to their use of alcohol and drugs, including opiates and cannabis. As you will see, a substantial proportion of the studies we will look at cite "substance abuse" and not just "alcohol abuse" as their target. The results of these studies will speak for themselves, but in general, treatments—including Twelve Step-based ones—have been found to work for the polysubstance abuser.

I will be discussing Project MATCH and its findings more in the chapters ahead, because it yielded a veritable treasure trove of valuable information relevant to some of the questions that will be addressed here about AA and how it works. Perhaps equally important, this landmark study helped spur more of the very kind of research that the Institute of Medicine was calling for. The intervening decades have seen a groundswell of new and intense interest in studying the Twelve Step program of AA through rigorous scientific research. That research, in turn, allowed this book to become a reality. Indeed, this emerging body of research sheds light not only on *whether* the AA program works, but on *how it works*. We will explore that research in depth here; my sources can be found in the references and sources section for those who wish to delve deeper into the details or simply to verify what is written here.

Though the information I present here is based soundly in research, my goal has been to write this book using nontechnical, jargon-free language as much as possible. As important and enlightening as it is, much of the research on the science of Twelve Step recovery lies in academic journals that are largely inaccessible (and incomprehensible) to anyone who has not been immersed in research design and statistical analysis. That is, of course, the general reading public, which remains to this day almost completely unaware of these important findings. Little wonder, then, that it has proven difficult to stand up for Twelve Step recovery in the face of its critics. My goal—armed with facts—is to do just that: to stand for the Twelve Step model in the face of long-standing and unchallenged criticism and skepticism, much of which is not based in fact.

It is my hope that members of AA will find the evidence I present here relevant and insightful with respect to their own recovery. Equally important, it is my hope that all those men and women who may be on the fence about going to an AA meeting—people who know they need help but who are hesitating based on criticism of the program—will benefit from learning about the *science* (as opposed to the myths) of Twelve Step recovery, and take that first step.

◆

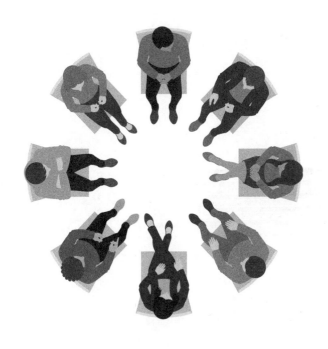

PART 1
It Works

From the Horse's Mouth

What AA's Membership Surveys Tell Us

Alcoholics Anonymous is a fellowship. It is not an academic institution; neither is it an organization in the traditional sense. In fact, AA intentionally lacks a formal hierarchy. If anything, AA is a bottom-up as opposed to a top-down fellowship. AA World Services does operate a General Services Office, with a professional staff and board of directors, but the purpose of that office is primarily informational. As defined in the AA Service Manual, "It serves as a clearinghouse and exchange point for the wealth of A.A. experience accumulated over the years, coordinates a wide array of activities and services, and oversees the publication, all translations of, and distribution of A.A. Conference approved literature and service materials." It does not set policy for individual groups, nor does it create or enforce any dogma that its constituents must commit to.

AA groups are guided by the basic texts, *Alcoholics Anonymous* and *Twelve Steps and Twelve Traditions*. The heart of AA lies not in any central office but in its meetings, which are run in accordance with long-standing rituals and traditions. Meetings are organized and run by those who attend them. This decentralization has allowed AA to evolve and adapt to the point where it has been referred to by Robin Room of the Alcohol Research Group in Berkeley, California, as an international "social movement." Today one can go to the main AA website (www.AA.org) and find a wide diversity of meeting types in addition to the traditional ones (speaker meetings and Step meetings, open meetings and closed meetings). The Seventh Tradition states, "Every A.A. group ought to be fully self-supporting, declining outside contributions," so that AA is sustained financially by donations from its membership, which again serves the interest of decentralization and diversity.

How AA Communicates

AA communicates to the world through its General Services Office, which operates a website, posts a national listing of meetings, and publishes a number of books (both print and ebook), pamphlets, booklets, DVDs, and audio CDs. All of this material is intended to be informative and consistent with AA principles and traditions. Most are available for free to people who can't afford them or are sold at a nominal cost. Authorship is either anonymous or limited to a first name and last name initial, the traditional means of identification in meetings to preserve anonymity. AA does not advertise; rather, it simply makes these materials available to those who seek them out. One will never see a television ad or billboard promoting AA (at least not one that is paid for by AA).

At its core level—the meeting—formal organization is minimal and largely determined by those who attend regularly. As stated in the Third Tradition, "The only requirement for A.A. membership is a desire to stop drinking." Groups usually register with the General Services Office so that other alcoholics can find them, but that is optional and they receive no direction from that office. Typically, members take turns volunteering for roles such as the meeting leader, secretary, and treasurer. Likewise the agenda for a meeting is determined by its members. Some meetings are open to a diversity of formats (speaker, Step discussion, and so on) whereas others, by mutual agreement, devote themselves to one consistent format.

Certain "rules of the road" are observed by tradition and are central to the AA culture. These include, first and foremost, anonymity. Examples of other rules include welcoming any newcomers to a meeting and not interrupting someone who is speaking or commenting on what anyone shares ("no cross talk").

One consequence of the AA culture as described above is that it does not engage those who criticize it. AA is content to remain a "program of attraction," in contrast to a "program of promotion," and it deliberately avoids getting involved in public controversies—including whether or not its Twelve Step program works. For that reason alone, AA has never taken part in or sponsored the kind of formal research on its effectiveness that comprises the bulk of material to be presented here. Although its members firmly believe in the effectiveness of the Twelve Step program, from its perspective every individual is free to take (or leave) AA. This lack of interchange with its critics may be exasperating for people who dislike AA and its Twelve Steps, but it has worked just fine for those who consider themselves members of the fellowship as well as those who may no longer attend meetings but who attribute their recovery and sobriety to their experience in the fellowship.

AA Membership Surveys

About the closest thing to "research" that AA has engaged in are its triennial membership surveys, which began in 1977. Consistent with AA tradition, these surveys are completed voluntarily by men and women who are currently attending AA meetings. No other conditions for participation are set. For example, a person does not have to attend a certain number of meetings per week, have a sponsor, or meet any other requirement in order to complete a survey. Rather, the AA central office randomly selects a certain number of groups from its listing of registered groups in the United States and sends them a number of surveys, hoping to get back about twenty completed surveys per group. Although it is more likely that a person who attends meetings regularly will be there when the surveys arrive, the surveys themselves ask about frequency of meeting attendance as well as a number of other AA-related activities. That information in turn can be correlated with other facts, such as how long the individual states that he or she has been sober.

No surveying method is perfect but it seems clear that AA's periodic member surveys seek to gather basic information that can then be shared. One of the limitations of the AA member surveys, however, is that they are limited to groups that choose to register themselves with AA's General Services Office. As of 2011, there were some 114,000 such groups worldwide. However, as many AA members know, certain groups choose not to register with AA. So it remains an unknown whether these groups would yield similar or divergent results.

It's worth considering the results of AA's member surveys, in particular to see what they can tell us about AA from the time of its first survey to the present. Later on we will examine patterns in the surveys from 1977 through 1989. For now, let's look at the most recent surveys: those reported in 2007 and 2011. AA organizes these survey results so that they can be easily understood. Here are some of the highlights.

Gender

In 2007, 67 percent of AA members were men and 33 percent were women. By comparison, in 2011, 65 percent were men and 35 percent were women. It appears, then, that a fellowship founded by men (and attended mainly by men) has not remained so. This trend, which was refleced in earlier surveys, had led one researcher, Linda Beckman, to the following conclusion after reviewing a number of surveys and studies on gender and recovery:

> When I started out on the journey of discovery involved in writing this paper, as a feminist I probably would have agreed with Jean Kirkpatrick that women who have feelings of inadequacy, worthlessness, and powerlessness and are faced with different issues than men need same-sex support groups that emphasize competence and self-efficacy, not powerlessness and humility. But having reviewed the literature and learned more about the processes of change in AA, I am much less confident about these conclusions. I now believe that AA, a fellowship originally designed by and composed primarily of men, appears to be equally or more effective for women than for men.

That's a rather startling statement from an academic teacher and researcher who admittedly started out with a bias in line with the writings of Jean Kirkpatrick, the founder of the organization Women for Sobriety. But it would appear that AA's decentralization has allowed it to evolve in ways that have attracted significant numbers of women. It is very possible to skim the AA meeting list in almost any area or region and find men's meetings and women's meetings for those who prefer that format. Alternatively, many men and women elect to include a same-sex meeting in their "mix" of meetings or choose a same-sex meeting as their "home group," a meeting they commit to attending regularly.

How They Got There

The triennial surveys also ask respondents to indicate how they were first introduced to AA. Here are those results:

Method of Introduction	2007	2011
Another AA member	33%	34%
A treatment facility	33%	32%
Self-motivated	31%	29%
Family	24%	25%
Court order	11%	12%
Counselor	8%	7%
Health professional	7%	7%

What is interesting about the above is how consistent the statistics are. About one in three people appear to have found AA on their own. Treatment facilities, counselors, and other health professionals together accounted for nearly half of the reasons given for trying AA. Also of significance: two out of three AA members reported that they sought counseling of some sort *in addition to AA* after they started attending meetings. This was true for both surveys. The significance of this data will emerge later when we look at actual research studies.

Age and Race

In 2007, 28 percent of AA members were under age forty and 64 percent were between forty and seventy. By 2011 these figures had changed only slightly: 26 percent were under forty, and 66 percent were between forty and seventy.

In the United States, 85 percent and 87 percent of AA members identified themselves as white in 2007 and 2011 respectively, strongly suggesting that AA is a fellowship that attracts primarily Caucasians. However, earlier research conducted by Klaus Makela of the Finnish Foundation for Alcohol Studies offers a somewhat different perspective. After surveying the growth of AA over time, Makela drew the following conclusion:

> Temperance cultures [primarily the U.S. and Canada] accounted for 60% of the membership of AA in 1986. The trends over time, however, point in a different direction. The share of all active AA groups in English-speaking and Scandinavian Protestant countries diminished from 1965 to 1986 while the share in central and southern European and particularly Latin American countries substantially increased.

If the trend identified by Makela continued beyond 1986, it is reasonable to assume that the racial composition of AA—at least outside of the United States—has become more diverse.

Correlates of Recovery

The title and theme of this book—*If You Work It, It Works!*—is quite intentional. It does not purport to present evidence about how AA and its Twelve Step program affects those who choose not to use it. In that regard, it is relevant to point out that about half of the men and women who come to AA remain active in the fellowship less than three months. Why these individuals stop going to meetings, and what happens to them afterward in terms of drinking, is unknown, as AA does not research the dynamics of these decisions, nor could it effectively survey anonymous members who have dropped out. In my own clinical practice, however, I have found that the motivations are diverse. They can include feeling uncomfortable for one reason or another at meetings. For some people, for example, severe social anxiety is a barrier. Others have expressed fears that, despite the AA commitment to anonymity, they would somehow be "outed" as alcoholics with resultant negative effects on their careers or social status. Or a single uncomfortable experience may be enough to turn an already ambivalent person away.

There are also some who simply cannot find it within themselves to identify with others at the meetings; they have the "I'm not that bad" or the "I can't relate to those people" syndrome. Finally, some men and women are turned off by the spiritual aspect of AA, in particular its references to "God as we understood Him" and a "Higher Power." Bill Wilson, a co-founder of AA and a lifelong agnostic, chose that language deliberately so as to open the AA door to a diversity of beliefs. Nevertheless, the mere mention of God or anything spiritual sends some people running for the nearest exit.

The bottom line is that the AA surveys can tell us what seems to be important to the men and women who do go to meetings. Here are some of the basics on the AA survey respondents:

Statistical factor	2007	2011
Years sober:		
Less than 1 year	31%	27%
1 to 5 years	24%	24%
5 to 10 years	12%	12%
More than 10 years	33%	36%
Average number of meetings attended per week	2.4	2.6
Percent who have a "home group"	86%	86%
Percent who have a sponsor	79%	81%

Let's take a look at the numbers above to see what we can learn from them. Again, we must keep in mind that these are data obtained from men and women who acknowledge that they are "working it." First, 72 percent of this group has been sober for more than a year, and a third have been sober for more than ten years. How did they manage to achieve that? Well, it would appear that one answer might be connected to *how* they work it. It would seem that, if you want to quit drinking and stay quit, you should aim for the following:

- Attend at least two and preferably three meetings a week.
- Choose a home group.
- Get a sponsor.

As we turn to controlled research on AA, we will see if the above prescription works and, if so, how well.

A Historical Perspective

One thing that stands out in the data presented above is its consistency. Moreover, it is steady not just from 2007 to 2011, but all the way back to 1977 when AA conducted its first membership survey. In 1989, for example, the average duration of sobriety reported by AA members was a little more than four years, and almost 30 percent had been sober between one and five years. Participants reported attending an average of three meetings per week; 80 percent said they had a sponsor, and 85 percent had a home group.

Of the above categories, the last two come up the most when I talk with people in recovery. They often point out, for example, that "All meetings are not created equal," meaning that they have found some meetings to be much better than others. This acknowledgment can be particularly helpful for newcomers who may be reticent to even try AA and more likely to stop going if they encounter a single bad meeting experience. Similarly, men and women with sustained recovery invariably stress that not only should newcomers get a temporary sponsor as soon as possible, but that they also need to be sure they feel comfortable with that person.

The kind of consistency reported in AA's member surveys is remarkable and suggests that at its core the culture of AA, including the derived wisdom that drives it, has remained remarkably stable over time. In particular, the levels of active participation in AA revealed in these statistics seem to be reasonable goals for a person who wants to stop drinking.

The information obtained through the triennial membership surveys has gradually changed in one dramatic way, and that has to do with drug abuse. In 1977 less than 20 percent of respondents reported being addicted to drugs in addition to alcohol. By 1989 that figure had climbed to nearly 45 percent. This appears to be another way in which AA has evolved over time. While some meetings choose to remain "orthodox," welcoming only fellow alcoholics, most meetings will typically include a mix of individuals—some with only a drinking problem, others with both a drinking and drug use problem. Similarly, whereas people who attended meetings a few decades ago might routinely be advised against taking any medications for mental illnesses, including those that were prescribed for them—thinking this could be another addiction—today many AA members freely admit to and are supported within the Twelve Step community for taking medications to treat conditions such as anxiety, depression, bipolar disorder, and post-traumatic stress disorder. AA World Services published a pamphlet affirming that members who take prescribed psychiatric medications have not relapsed, and by and large, attitudes among group members have changed dramatically and now generally accept medications prescribed to treat psychiatric disorders.

Summing Up

We start our investigation into the science of Twelve Step recovery through the lens of what men and women in AA have to say about themselves. Some might contend that this is biased: that active AA members are motivated to paint a rosy picture of the program. But this argument would mean that self-reported data have been systematically falsified since 1977—a hard claim to swallow. A better explanation is that the AA membership surveys tell us, from the horse's mouth as it were, what the men and women who choose to work the program do that enables it to work for them.

Now let's turn to another lens and examine what we know about the Twelve Step program and recovery as viewed from the outside—by academic researchers who have studied those who choose AA and how it affects them.

Food for Thought

1. Have any of the factors talked about in this chapter—such as doubts about whether Twelve Step meetings really work, one bad experience at meeting, or gender issues—prevented you from attending a meeting in the past? What's preventing you now from giving it a try?

2. If you currently attend Twelve Step meetings, how many do you attend per week? After reading this chapter, do you think it would be helpful to attend more?

3. Do you have a home group? A sponsor? If not, what is preventing you from choosing a home group or finding a sponsor?

◆

The View from Outside

AA and Recovery

Now let's examine what researchers have found when they have turned their spotlights on AA's Twelve Step program and how involvement in AA relates to staying sober.

When approaching the concept of "recovery," academic researchers look at several outcome variables. One thing they always consider is abstinence: how many days a person does not drink. When converted to a percentage, this measure is called percent days abstinent, or PDA. Researchers are also interested in how much a person drinks when he or she does drink. Therefore, they often also ask for information on drinks per drinking day, or DDD. Whether they are evaluating the effectiveness of a treatment for alcohol use disorders or assessing what happens to people who attend AA, researchers routinely look at both PDA and DDD. Accordingly, you will encounter these terms repeatedly throughout this book.

A second factor to keep in mind when we explore research on recovery is that the vast majority of studies on AA and its effectiveness have involved men and women who were diagnosed with an *alcohol use disorder,* the term the American Psychiatric Association now uses to cover both alcohol abuse and dependence in the newest edition of their *Diagnostic and Statistical Manual of Mental Disorders* (5th ed.; *DSM-5*). In other words, these individuals are *not* low-risk (or "social") drinkers who may have a glass or two of wine, or a beer or two, a few times a week. Their self-reported drinking habits involve much more alcohol consumption than that. Furthermore, almost all those who become involved in research do so after seeking help in one form or another.

"Naturalistic" Studies

The first research method we will examine is used in studies that follow men and women who do (or don't) choose to participate in AA. Rudolf and Bernice Moos conducted one such study. Rudolf Moos is a professor in the Department of Psychiatry and Behavioral Sciences at Stanford University and the recipient of the Hofheimer Prize Award from the *Journal of Psychiatric Research.* He and his wife and co-researcher, Bernice, are both affiliated with the Center for Health Care Evaluation, also in Palo Alto, California.

This study began by identifying a sample of 362 men and women who had experienced enough problems related to drinking that they were motivated to call an information and referral center to find help. They were diagnosed based on what they reported about themselves and their drinking via a questionnaire. The researchers then followed these volunteers for sixteen years—a remarkable length of time for any study—assessing them periodically.

The Moos sample was divided into three categories, depending on what individuals chose to do. No one was assigned to any of these groups; rather, they simply represent the different pathways that the participants voluntarily chose in the first year of the study. That is what makes this a *naturalistic* study. Here are the pathways:

- *Group 1:* People who decided to start going to AA but not to seek professional treatment of any kind

- *Group 2:* People who decided to start going to AA and seek professional treatment *at the same time*

- *Group 3:* People who decided to seek professional treatment but did not start going to AA

When examined "at the starting gate"—when they first entered this long-term study—the three groups did not differ demographically or in terms of their drinking patterns. For example, those with the worst drinking problems did not systematically choose one path over the others. This is important because it means that initially the three groups were essentially alike other than for the different pathways they chose.

All three groups were followed for sixteen years and assessed after years one, three, eight, and finally again at year sixteen. This is indeed a long time to follow a group of people and is a good example of what researchers call a *longitudinal* study. Another example of a naturalistic study would be to identify two comparable groups of people, one that then decided to diet and exercise carefully, and a second that did not. Assuming that the two groups were equivalent at the outset, a longitudinal study could be used to compare the status of their health one year, three years, eight years, and sixteen years later.

Obviously, naturalistic longitudinal studies have the potential to tell us a lot about the consequences of pursuing different pathways. In the case of the Moos study, here is what they found:

- People in group 2, who opted for treatment and AA at the same time, participated in AA longer and more frequently. Moreover, people in this group were the most likely to stay sober throughout the course of the study.

- People who began attending AA but then dropped out were more likely to start drinking again.

- The longer people remained active in AA, the more likely they were to stay sober at all four follow-ups: one year, three years, eight years, and sixteen years.

One additional finding of interest in this study concerned those in group 3, who opted at the outset for treatment but decided against going to AA. Some of the men and women in this group later decided to try AA, but this delayed move did not seem to improve their chances of staying sober. We do know, however, that when they finally decided to attend AA meetings, they did so less often than those in the other groups. The authors conjecture the men and women in group 3 may have held more negative or skeptical attitudes about AA; for example, that it encourages dependency. Alternatively, they may not have believed (rightly or wrongly) that their alcohol use disorder was severe enough to warrant attending AA. Either way, these late-starters did not fare as well as their counterparts who opted either for AA alone or AA plus treatment from the beginning of their recovery efforts.

A companion naturalistic longitudinal study, also conducted by researchers at the Center for Health Care Evaluation, followed 135 individuals (half men, half women) who also reached out to an information and referral service in Northern California. Prior to initiating these contacts, none of the men and women had ever received treatment for an alcohol use disorder.

The researchers followed this group for three years, gathering information at different points in time. Here are some of the questions they sought to answer:

- How severe was each individual's drinking problem?
- Had they sought treatment after making contact?
- Had they tried AA?
- Were they drinking heavily, moderately, or not at all at each point in time?
- How much support did they feel they had for staying sober from a spouse, friends, or family?
- What was their socioeconomic status?

One thing I found of interest in this particular study, which was published in a 1995 edition of the journal *Addictive Behaviors*, was a footnote that appeared on the first page. The footnote addresses whether recovery that is associated with attending AA should be considered "natural" or a "treatment." I believe the authors correctly asserted that AA is not a treatment, for two reasons. First, they suggest that fellowships like AA are better viewed as natural *community resources and ways of life*, rather than treatments.

Second, self-help, peer recovery fellowships like AA require no professional guidance or intervention, but are run by their members. This is important, because critics of AA often refer to it as an "unproven treatment," when in fact AA has always considered itself to be a recovery fellowship, not a treatment program. That's not to say, however, that AA and the Twelve Step program is "unproven" as a way to stop drinking. That is the very issue we are examining here.

Out of this starting group of 135 men and women with alcohol use disorders, 28 eventually became abstinent—they did not drink at all, showed no objective signs of dependency, and had no drinking-related problems. Another 29 people in the study ended up being "moderate" drinkers—they drank significantly less, showed a few (but not a lot) objective signs of dependency, and reported few drinking-related problems. This finding, that some people became moderate drinkers, will be addressed in more detail in the next chapter. For now, let's explore what the researchers discovered when they took a closer look at the people who abstained:

- This group had *more severe* drinking problems at the outset.
- They believed their drinking was a *very serious* problem.
- They had *little social support*; instead *they relied heavily on AA to maintain their recovery.*

The second bullet may be the most significant. These individuals had decided on their own that they had a severe drinking problem that needed attention. In other words, they agreed with the diagnosis they received. Findings from this second naturalistic study echo those from the one previously discussed, but they also amplify them. These additional data point in a specific direction: the men and women in this study who had more severe drinking problems, who believed their problem was severe, and who reported having little social support *were inclined to choose AA as their solution.* It became their path to recovery, and they became abstinent. Moreover, they did so without any outside intervention.

In contrast to the above, the group whose problems were less severe, and who reported having the added benefit of supportive relationships, eventually became moderate drinkers. Again, this does not mean that they experienced no drinking-related problems, but rather that they experienced relatively few of them.

These results raise the question of whether abstinence or moderate drinking should be the goal of treatment, and this will be addressed in chapter 4. As it stands, the two naturalistic studies we've looked at so far support the idea that AA works for those who choose to work it. In addition, and perhaps because AA has become so ubiquitous and accessible in society, it is often chosen as a solution, especially for those with more severe drinking problems who do not have other sources of social support.

AA Following Treatment

A variation on naturalistic studies (which follow a group of problem drinkers even before they decide how to deal with it) are studies in which researchers investigate what happens to men and women *after* they initially receive treatment for their drinking problems. Although most alcohol treatment centers advocate AA attendance, there is a great deal of variability in just how energetically they do so—and some avoid taking a stance on AA altogether. With that in mind, it can be instructive to examine the trajectories of peoples' lives following treatment.

The first study we'll look at was the result of collaboration between researchers at the Veterans Administration Palo Alto Health Care System and Stanford University Medical Center. For two years this group followed 2,319 men who had been diagnosed as alcohol dependent (or, using current diagnostic terminology, having a severe alcohol use disorder) and subsequently received treatment through the VA health care system. They assessed these men at years one and two, measuring not only how much these men were drinking at each point in time, but also how many of the following negative drinking-related *consequences* they had experienced in each of these areas:

- *Health:* Health problems connected to alcohol abuse, such as diabetes and hypertension
- *Legal:* Arrests for DUI, domestic violence, and so on
- *Monetary:* Late credit card or rent payments, also often related to alcohol abuse
- *Occupational:* Lost jobs, poor performance evaluations
- *Interpersonal:* Marital or family conflict
- *Housing:* Eviction

The measure of *AA involvement* used in this study included how many meetings the men attended, how often they read AA material, how often they communicated with a sponsor, and how many AA friends they had. AA involvement, therefore, could range from not at all to very much.

Finally, the researchers assessed just how *motivated* these men were to seek treatment at the outset, *before* they even entered treatment, using a questionnaire that asked participants about their "readiness for change."

This study is of particular interest because of the last variable that the researchers included. Some people have argued that AA only benefits those who are highly motivated to seek it out. Many also assume—explicitly or implicitly—that these people do so reluctantly and only after their drinking causes them to "hit bottom," meaning suffering severe consequences. One could argue that this would be just fine with AA, which, as we've said, has deliberately chosen to remain a program of attraction, not promotion. Still, it would be interesting to gain some insight into just how important that initial motivation factor is.

Here is what these researchers found:

- Greater AA involvement was linked with decreased drinking and fewer drinking-related consequences.

- AA participation levels and better outcomes were evident regardless of whether these men had prior experience with AA.

- AA participation and better outcomes did not depend on having a more severe or a less severe drinking problem.

- Motivation prior to treatment did *not* predict level of AA involvement or degree of drinking-related consequences.

These researchers did not report how many men remained completely abstinent throughout the two-year study. Instead, like AA itself, which emphasizes "progress over perfection," they focused on whether AA involvement was enough to explain significant improvements in drinking and its consequences. They concluded that it was. The most significant outcome of this study was evidence that *greater involvement in AA was associated with significant decreases in drinking as well as in negative consequences associated with drinking.* Now let's look at some of the other results.

The last finding would appear to contradict the notion that only highly motivated individuals will benefit from AA. However, although "readiness for change" did not predict outcome here, the authors of the study point out that motivation is a *dynamic*, not a *static* thing. In short, people's motivation can *change*, often depending on circumstances. I have encountered more than a few individuals whose experience attests to this. These are men and women who have told me that they attended AA meetings for some time before ever seeing that they actually needed it and that they needed to pursue abstinence as opposed to moderate drinking. This is in line with the advice that an AA sponsor may offer to a skeptical newcomer: "Fake it 'til you make it." In other words, put your doubts aside and act as if you need to stay clean and sober.

In this case, if motivation at the beginning of treatment did not predict AA involvement or drinking-related consequences after treatment, perhaps treatment itself, along with exposure to AA, increased that motivation along the way for a significant proportion of these men. Their goal for themselves may have changed as a result of going to AA meetings. We will explore this issue of personal goals and how they relate to recovery more closely later on.

Another significant finding from this study is that the severity of a man's drinking problem at the beginning of the study did not predict how well he would do over the two years. Although all of the men in this study did have significant drinking problems, the severity nevertheless varied. This finding means, then, that participating in AA helped both those men with the most severe drinking problems *and* those with less severe drinking problems. This, too, runs counter to the popular stereotype that AA is only for those men and women who have "hit bottom" as a result of drinking.

The *Journal of Substance Abuse Treatment,* in 2014, reported on the results of an ambitious nine-year study of how attendance at Twelve Step meetings following treatment for an alcohol use disorder related to recovery. This study is important to consider for a number of reasons, the first being its comprehensiveness. A total of 1,945 men and women who underwent outpatient or inpatient treatment were recruited for the study. This large group was then assessed one year, five years, seven years, and nine years following treatment. They reported on how frequently they attended Twelve Step meetings and how much and how often they drank, and their self-reported behaviors were validated by random urine screening.

This study is important for a second reason: it represented a collaborative effort between an academic institution and the Kaiser Permanente Health Care System, a large nonprofit health care provider. These participants, significantly, were all men and women who had health insurance that covered their treatment. In effect, this was a sample of middle-class Americans who decided they needed help with a drinking (or drug) problem.

This group of men and women found their way into treatment via different pathways: through medical providers at Kaiser Permanente, through employee assistance programs, and through their own initiative. During treatment they were required to attend at least one Twelve Step meeting a week, but after treatment they were on their own. Twelve Step groups included AA, but participants could also choose to attend Narcotics Anonymous (NA) or Cocaine Anonymous (CA), both of which were available in that geographic area. While AA focuses exclusively on recovery from alcoholism, both NA and CA apply the Twelve Step program to recovery from any mood-altering substance.

Also unique to this study was the way the researchers analyzed the data they collected. Without getting too complex, essentially they were able to uncover not only whether AA attendance over time was predictive of recovery, but also whether the reverse might be true. In other words, they could determine whether it was the Twelve Step fellowship that promoted abstinence or whether being clean and sober actually caused people to go to meetings. Here is what they found:

> Our time-lagged results showed that greater 12 step meeting attendance led to increases in 5-year abstinence and to a lesser extent in 7-year abstinence.

Causal associations in the reverse direction were not detected for those years.

These results make it clear that sobriety itself doesn't somehow make a person get involved in AA or another Twelve Step fellowship; rather, getting involved in a fellowship is what leads to recovery. The authors finish with this comment:

> Importantly our analysis extends findings to a diverse population of treatment seekers, namely men and women with alcohol and drug use disorders who were insured members of an integrated health care organization.

This last comment is noteworthy because it further debunks the long-standing stereotype about AA—that it is only for those who are "down and out" and who have "bottomed out." The people in this study were neither; they were living and working in middle-class America. They were not panhandling, sleeping under bridges, eating at soup kitchens, or living in shelters.

The next study we'll turn to was conducted by researchers led by Dr. Lee Ann Kaskutas of the Alcohol Research Group and the University of California. They recruited 349 men and women (35 percent were women) from ten public and private alcohol treatment programs. While these individuals' drinking problems were serious enough to qualify them for treatment, once again they did vary in severity. This group—who had never before undergone treatment for drinking problems—were then assessed one year, three years, and five years after finishing treatment. At each point in time they were asked how often they'd had a drink in the previous thirty days. This is a measure of drinking behavior frequently used by researchers, especially when study participants are to be reassessed on several different occasions. And it makes sense. If an individual consistently reports, at several points in time, that he or she has been clean and sober for the previous thirty days, that can indicate that the individual's recovery is going well. Accordingly, people who report no drinks in the prior thirty days are classified as *abstinent* (at the time they are assessed); those who report having consumed even a single drink in that time period are classified as *non-abstinent*.

As with the study described above, these researchers were interested in seeing how much this group of men and women had used AA, and how that related to their recovery. The participants were divided into groups, as follows:

- *Low AA involvement:* This group mainly attended AA only during the first year after finishing treatment.

- *Medium AA involvement:* This group continued to attend AA meetings, at an average rate of sixty meetings per year after completing treatment.

- *High AA involvement:* This group also continued to attend AA meetings after treatment, but at a rate of two hundred or more meetings per year.

- *Declining AA involvement:* This group was like the high-involvement group for the first year following treatment, but by the fifth year they were attending on average only six meetings per year.

These groups make for some interesting comparisons, as the researchers assessed their rates of abstinence for the preceding thirty days at numerous points: one, three, and five years following treatment.

The results of the five-year follow-up assessments were striking:

- 43 percent of the low-involvement group were abstinent at each of the three follow-up assessments (years one, three, and five).

- About two-thirds of those in the medium-involvement group were abstinent at the year-one follow-up, and this increased to 79 percent at the year-five follow-up.

- 86 percent of the high-involvement group were abstinent at the year-one follow-up, but this leveled off at 79 percent by the time of the five-year follow-up.

- 79 percent of the declining group were abstinent at the year-one follow-up, but this declined to 60 percent at the five-year follow-up.

The conclusion here is clear and unmistakable: greater involvement in AA is associated with better long-term outcomes for men and women initially diagnosed as having a severe alcohol disorder. Declining involvement, meanwhile, is associated with declining abstinence. However, in this sample at least, the added gain from attending two hundred or more meetings versus sixty AA meetings a year did not make the same impact as extending attendance at the medium involvement level beyond the first year after treatment. This is another slant on what it means to "work" the AA program. It would appear that to maximize one's chances of staying clean and sober, a person's best bet is to remain continuously and steadily active in a Twelve Step fellowship at a rate of or above sixty meetings a year.

Another result of this study that I found interesting is that when asked at year five, over half of those in the declining group said they still felt like they were a *member* of AA. In other words, they still *identified* with AA, even though they were attending fewer meetings. It is plausible to conjecture, then, that these men and women had internalized much of the program's wisdom during their days of greater involvement in AA. A majority of this group was doing well, albeit less well than their peers who were more active in the program.

Let's turn now to some research studies led by Christine Timko, PhD. Timko is with the Center for Health Care Evaluation in Palo Alto, California, where she holds the position of Research Career Scientist. Timko completed her doctorate in social psychology at the University of Massachusetts and a postdoctoral fellowship in health psychology from Yale University.

In this first study, 345 men were followed for six months after they completed a voluntary outpatient treatment program for an alcohol use disorder. The researchers were, of course, interested in how this group fared in terms of drinking, so they assessed how often and how much they drank over these six months. Again, those who had not used any alcohol or drugs during the preceding thirty days were classified as *abstinent*; any use of alcohol or drugs meant they were classified as *non-abstinent*. Also assessed was how *severe* the alcohol use disorder was before treatment.

Aside from drinking behavior per se, Timko and her colleagues were interested in looking at a number of additional factors to determine how each of them might relate to drinking behavior. So they explored the following:

- *Demographics:* Age, race, education, and income of the participants
- *Religious practices:* How often each person reported praying, meditating, or thinking about God
- *Extraversion:* How easy it is for people to initiate friendships or disclose information about themselves

- *AA involvement:* The belief that addiction is a disease that makes life "unmanageable," commitment to abstinence, attending meetings, "working the Twelve Steps," having a sponsor

This group's first finding was that extraversion was associated with attending more AA meetings—in effect, being naturally outgoing is an asset when it comes to getting active in a Twelve Step fellowship. This makes intuitive sense, as shy individuals would need to overcome or at least moderate that shyness in order to become involved in AA—and sometimes just to get through the door to their first meeting! In this regard, AA's admonishment that "the most important member at a meeting is the newcomer" may be important for existing AA members to keep in mind. Offering a warm and accepting welcome to a shy newcomer might make all the difference for that person's recovery.

In addition, these researchers learned that having a *less stable residence plus more religious practices* was associated with greater AA involvement. Involvement means more than merely attending meetings, so it appears that AA appealed to those whose home lives were less stable and who held some form of religious beliefs. In a way this also makes sense, as it could make the phrase "God as we understood Him" in the Third Step of AA less off-putting to this particular group of men and women.

Finally, the data in this study suggested that men with less education attended more AA meetings than men with higher levels of education. However, in this particular case the phrase "less education" should be taken in context, as the study participants reported completing an average of thirteen years of education, which is actually fairly high.

Now, as for actually staying sober, here are the factors that predicted abstinence:

- more *attendance* at AA meetings
- greater *involvement* in AA
- greater *acceptance* of Twelve Step beliefs

So, what lessons can we draw from this study? Well, it would appear that being extraverted (as opposed to socially shy) and also having some spiritual beliefs, facilitates going to meetings and getting involved. Overall, however, it is involvement itself and acceptance of AA beliefs that predict sobriety most strongly. The first of these is a behavioral factor: being there, as it were. The second factor is more of a cognitive or even spiritual factor, having to do not as much with what a person *does*, as much as what that person *believes*. The bottom line, then, is that action combined with belief predicts recovery.

In a related study with the same group of 345 men, Timko and associates explored what would happen if these men, as they entered treatment, randomly received either a *standard referral* to AA versus an *intensive referral* to AA. Those who were assigned to the standard referral treatment were given a schedule of AA and NA meetings in the area. The therapist encouraged each man to go to AA, NA, or both. But that was the extent of their "AA referral."

This level of referral to Twelve Step fellowships, incidentally, is fairly typical. Many treatment centers will assert that their programs are "Twelve Step based" or "Twelve Step friendly" and that they support the use of AA and NA as an adjunct to treatment. That may be true, but it is often left to the individual clinicians to decide how far to go in encouraging or facilitating involvement in these fellowships. For many therapists, this standard referral—providing a meeting list (or a website address) and recommending AA or NA—is sufficient.

In the intensive referral treatment arm of the study, in contrast, therapists went much further in encouraging involvement in a Twelve Step fellowship. In the first session, for example, the therapist not only gave the patient a listing of AA and NA meetings but went over the list, pointing out meetings that other patients said they liked, and even offered directions on finding the meeting location. The patient was then given a handout that described what the patient could expect when going to a meeting, including how meetings were organized, what the rules of the road were, and what a home group and sponsor were.

Next, and again in this first session, the therapist would place a call to an active AA or NA member (men and women who were involved in AA and/or NA and who had volunteered to participate) and arrange for that person to meet the patient ahead of a meeting and then attend it together. Finally, if the patient had not attended an AA or NA meeting at the time of the second session, the therapist repeated this process of contacting an AA/NA volunteer.

The entire group (standard referral and intensive referral) was assessed six months later for alcohol and drug use, as well as for how often participants attended Twelve Step meetings and how involved they were in AA or NA. Alcohol and drug use was assessed using a diagnostic interview: the Addiction Severity Index, or ASI. Twelve Step fellowship involvement included things like reading Twelve Step literature (such as *Alcoholics Anonymous*), doing service work (such as setting up chairs or making coffee), having a sponsor, and so on.

Clearly, the intensive referral approach was intended to go much further than simply recommending AA or NA. It aimed to educate patients about Twelve Step fellowships and to facilitate and promote their early involvement in them. The results they reported, after six months, are instructive. First, during that six-month period, patients who received the intensive referral did not differ so much from those who received the standard referral in terms of how many Twelve Step fellowship meetings they attended. Specifically, those who received the intensive referral attended an average of sixty-four meetings over the six months, as compared to fifty-seven for the standard referral group.

But despite having attended roughly the same number of meetings, the men who received the intensive referral *improved more with respect to their alcohol and other drug use* over the six months than the men in the standard referral group. This leads to the logical question: why the difference?

As it turns out, the difference had to do with involvement. For example, the men in the intensive referral group were much more likely to have done service work at meetings. They were also more likely to have read from the AA "Big Book" (*Alcoholics Anonymous*), the "Twelve and Twelve" (*Twelve Steps and Twelve Traditions*), or other AA and NA publications. In addition, they were more likely to report having a sponsor or even being a sponsor. Finally, more of them reported having had the "spiritual awakening" that AA believes can come from earnestly working the Twelve Steps. In sum, the men who received the intensive referral were not necessarily attending more AA or NA meetings but were identifying with and more involved in one or both of those fellowships than the men who had received the standard referral.

Let's look at another study that explored this issue of involvement. This study was reported in the *Journal of Substance Abuse*

Treatment and was conducted collaboratively by psychologists at the Harry S. Truman College and DePaul University in Chicago. They were interested in a concept they labeled *categorical Twelve Step involvement.* They used the following criteria to classify people as being categorically involved in a Twelve Step fellowship:

- They have a sponsor.
- They read Twelve Step literature.
- They do service work, such as making coffee, setting up meetings, or cleaning up afterward.
- They have at times called or otherwise contacted other fellowship members for help.

It would seem self-evident that being categorically involved in AA (or any Twelve Step fellowship) would mean that you identify yourself as a member of that fellowship. The aim of these researchers was to see if men and women who were categorically committed would fare better with respect to recovery in the long run, as compared to men and women who were not categorically committed.

To answer this question, the research team decided to compare individuals who completed an intensive but brief residential addiction treatment program and then were willing to go on to an aftercare program. They chose two such programs that had very different emphases. One was Oxford House, where participants could live while pursuing work. Oxford House strongly encourages Twelve Step involvement as defined above. The alternative aftercare program offered outpatient counseling but not housing. Therefore, this form of aftercare was not as immersed in Twelve Step culture and not as dedicated to Twelve Step recovery.

The next step was to recruit such a group of men and women who (1) had completed a residential addiction treatment program, and (2) were willing to be randomly assigned to one of these two different kinds of aftercare. It took them a year and a half to identify fifty-seven men and ninety-three women who met these criteria. Those who went to Oxford House spent an average of 256 days living there, while those assigned to the other aftercare had various living arrangements, including their own or their spouse's home, a family member's home, or even, in some cases, a shelter.

Both groups were followed closely and assessed two years after completing their residential treatment programs. What they found was in part what they predicted: *individuals who scored high on categorical commitment were significantly more likely to maintain continuous abstinence for the entire two years after treatment.* This finding once more casts important light on what "working" the Twelve Step program involves. Simultaneously, it points to the likely outcome if a person opts to not "work it" (or at least not as conscientiously).

The other finding of interest had to do with exposure to the Oxford House program. Those men and women who were most engaged in the Oxford House program were also more likely to remain abstinent for the two years than the participants who were less involved in the various AA-related activities it offered its residents. In other words, categorical commitment worked independently of simply living in an Oxford House.

The conclusion, then, is clear: being immersed in a Twelve Step program of recovery—not merely attending and completing a treatment program—is what leads to categorical commitment, and it is that commitment that seems most predictive of recovery. As a corollary, it's safe to say that what can be accomplished by sending someone to a treatment program depends in large measure on how much of the AA culture they choose to absorb (and follow through on) in the course of that treatment. To say that a person has "gone to rehab," in other words, means relatively little in and of itself. What matters more is what happened to that person both during and after treatment. Men and women who contemplate rehab must, therefore, be sure they see it not as a "cure" but as an opportunity to begin to alter their lifestyle in ways that will promote recovery.

This issue—of coming to identify oneself with a Twelve Step fellowship and how that identification in turn relates to recovery—was evident again in another study, this one conducted by a group of social psychologists at London South Bank University.

Social psychologists have long studied the way individuals choose to define themselves and how that identity in turn affects their behavior. In doing so, they have followed in the footsteps of Erik Erikson, whose seminal work *Identity: Youth and Crisis* first set forth the notion that the identity we embrace as we pass through adolescence represents a kind of psychological template or road map that strongly influences the direction our lives will take.

Social psychological research appears to support Erikson's contention, as it has focused attention on how deciding to identify with a particular group can relate to the person's physical or mental health. In one study, for example, researchers found that survivors of stroke who chose to identify themselves that way and attend ongoing support groups reported enhanced feelings of well-being as compared to stroke survivors who opted not to become active in such groups.

Using studies like this as a springboard, other researchers have investigated how identifying oneself as a "recovering alcoholic" (or "recovering addict") affects that person's well-being (as opposed to not embracing that identity). The researchers at London South Bank studied a group of men and women, all of whom were attending Alcoholics Anonymous or Narcotics Anonymous groups. They divided this group further based on how much each individual identified with the phrase *recovering alcoholic* (or recovering addict) versus simply an *alcoholic* (or addict). These two identities were measured by how strongly (on a scale of 1 to 7) each participant endorsed statements such as

- Being an AA (NA) member is a central part of who I am.
- I would describe myself as an AA (NA) member.

The higher the score, the more the individual identified as a recovering alcoholic or addict.

The researchers then assessed participants for their self-efficacy, which was measured by their responses (again on a scale of 1 to 7) to statements such as

- I can remain abstinent.
- I can manage my addiction.

Again, the higher the score, the more the individual is said to experience self-efficacy.

Here is what these researchers found:

- The more the individual identified as a recovering alcoholic or recovering addict (as opposed to just alcoholic or addict) the higher the person's level of self-efficacy.
- Higher self-efficacy was associated with more months clean and sober.
- The more individuals leaned toward the *recovering* identity, the less likely they were to report having relapsed

into drinking or drug use during the previous two years, as compared to those who identified themselves as simply alcoholics or addicts.

The above findings become even more interesting if we look back for a moment on the study by Lee Ann Kaskutas, mentioned earlier. If you recall, she grouped her participants into those who reported *low* AA attendance rates, *medium* attendance rates, and *high* attendance rates, and found that abstinence rates were highest for the group with the highest level of attendance (79 percent abstinent). However, Kaskutas also reported that 61 percent of those in a group that reported a declining rate of AA attendance were also abstinent. What is interesting, and perhaps relevant in light of the London South Bank study, is that over half of those in Kaskutas's declining group said that they still felt like they were "members" of AA. In other words, they *identified* with AA despite their falling attendance rates.

So, the evidence suggests that one factor influencing recovery has to do with not just whether a person attends AA (or NA) but with how much that person identifies with a Twelve Step fellowship. The evidence on "involvement" and how it relates to recovery also supports this concept of identity. It's reasonable, for example, to postulate that greater involvement in a fellowship signifies greater identification with that fellowship. Therefore, when assessing an individual's experience with a Twelve Step fellowship and what might arise due to that experience, it is not enough to simply ask if that person has attended AA or NA— or even how many meetings were attended. Rather, one needs to ask questions like, "Do you feel like you are a *member* of AA (or NA)?" or, "Do you think of yourself as a *recovering* alcoholic (or addict)?" The answers to these questions are likely to be pre-dictive. Individuals who merely attend meetings but do not iden-tify as program members could be said to be "on the outside, looking in," and their recovery may be less robust for it.

Summing Up

The research we've looked at in this chapter focused on the re-lationship between Twelve Step group affiliation and drinking. The primary measure used was abstinence, generally defined as not drinking at all over a stated period of time. That "affiliation," we learned, includes not only being there (going to meetings) but also how deeply involved an individual is within a Twelve Step fellowship. Most of these studies involved following men and women after they received some form of formal treatment for alcohol or drug dependence. What exactly that treatment con-sisted of may have varied, though in one case we looked at, the therapists made a deliberate and concerted effort to encourage AA or NA attendance.

One conclusion we can draw from these studies is that there is a significant correlation between AA or NA meeting atten-dance and recovery. Furthermore, when a therapist goes beyond simply recommending that a client go to AA or NA—for ex-ample, by suggesting specific meetings and even arranging for the client to meet a member of that fellowship—the outcome is even better.

These studies also showed us, however, that involvement is not necessarily the same thing as attendance at AA or any other support group. What goes on inside the individual also matters. Involvement is about identification. On this deeper level, involve-ment means saying things like "I am a recovering alcoholic," or "I admit that drinking has made my life unmanageable." It also

means doing things like getting a sponsor and actively participating in meetings. Finally, involvement also has a spiritual component, as measured by the correlation between recovery and
believing in some form of power greater than sheer individual
willpower.

Let us move on now to examine AA and its effectiveness as
assessed by studies in which the primary goal of treatment was to
facilitate involvement as defined above.

Food for Thought

1. Have you had doubts that complete abstinence from alcohol and other drug use is a realistic goal for you? What has caused those doubts?

2. Are any of the following barriers for you in attending or getting more involved in Twelve Step meetings? If so, what can you do to overcome them?

   a. age, race, education, or income

   b. religious beliefs or practices

   c. socialization skills or introversion

3. Do you identify as an AA, NA, or other Twelve Step group member? If not, are there things you can do to increase your involvement, such as attending more meetings, doing service work, calling other members for support, or reading more literature?

◆

Focused Therapies

Facilitating AA Involvement

In this chapter we will look at what happens when treatment does not simply recommend AA, but actually aims to achieve the following goals:

educate clients about AA—how meetings work, the AA "rules of the road," and so on

address and attempt to resolve any reservations clients may have about Twelve Step fellowships, such as that AA is a religion

help to reduce any emotional barriers to AA meeting involvement, such as social anxiety, and make AA attendance more comfortable

assist clients in "working" some of the Steps of AA

Timko's study on "intensive referral" that we cited in the previous chapter was a precursor in a way to the kinds of intervention we'll be looking at here. As outlined in the above goals, these therapies extend well beyond simply promoting AA attendance as an "adjunct" to treatment. Rather, what we are looking at here are therapies that seek to bring AA into the therapist's office, if you will, so that AA involvement is itself the focus of treatment.

We will take a close look at two therapies that have been tested via well-designed research—so-called random clinical trials— that social scientists consider the gold standard in determining if a treatment really works. In both cases, these focused treatments have been compared to other ("standard") treatment approaches with respect to their relative effectiveness. Keep in mind that while AA and its sister Twelve Step fellowships are not addiction treatment programs, and rather position themselves as voluntary peer recovery groups, what we will be looking at here are protocols designed for use in treatment programs conducted by trained professionals. Here are the two treatment approaches:

- Making Alcoholics Anonymous Easier (MAAEZ)
- Twelve Step Facilitation (TSF)

MAAEZ

Making Alcoholics Anonymous Easier, or MAAEZ, was designed by Lee Ann Kaskutas and Edward Oberste of the Alcohol Research Group in Berkeley, California. The stated goals of MAAEZ are as follows:

- to facilitate participation in Alcoholics Anonymous or in other Twelve Step programs such as Narcotics Anonymous
- to transition into the culture of Alcoholics Anonymous

MAAEZ is conducted in a group format over six sessions. There is an introductory session, which is basically about "what to expect" when going to an AA or NA meeting. In this session the therapists (assisted by "advanced" MAAEZ participants) share basic information about MAAEZ itself (use of first names only, subjects that will be covered in sessions, and so on). Participants also share basic information about themselves, such as their drug of choice and their history of prior treatment, if any. "Newcomers" are then given information about AA and its effectiveness as found through research, as well as information about the AA culture: the diversity of meetings, rituals and traditions, and so on. Meeting schedules are handed out and participants are asked to commit to attend an AA or NA meeting before the second MAAEZ session.

Other topics covered in MAAEZ sessions:

- *Spirituality:* Defines it not in terms of religious dogma but as "a way of living"

- *Principles not personalities:* Aims to debunk some of the more common misconceptions about AA, such as that it is a religious cult that indoctrinates or "brainwashes" its members

- *Sponsorship:* Explains the role of sponsorship within Twelve Step fellowships and helps participants identify what they would look for in a sponsor

- *Living sober:* Addresses the role and importance of lifestyle change in recovery

For the sixth MAAEZ session, the individual returns to an introductory session, only this time as a "graduate" of the program who now answers questions and supports program newcomers in their first steps toward recovery.

Each MAAEZ session ends with a homework assignment. These include assignments to read AA literature, attend AA meetings, get phone numbers and talk to other AA members, and ask someone to volunteer as a temporary sponsor.

It's important to note that the homework assignments that

are integral to MAAEZ, along with the contents of its sessions, mirror two things already revealed in our survey of research on AA. First, the goals of MAAEZ correspond to what AA members themselves say in membership surveys about their recovery practices. Those men and women who reported having sustained recovery, for example, were very likely to have sponsors, and three out of four who received some sort of counseling said that the counseling influenced their decision to attend AA meetings.

MAAEZ also encourages the very behaviors associated with greater AA involvement, an outcome that emerged from our review of the post-treatment recovery careers of men and women in the last chapter. These include things such as reading AA material, establishing friendships through AA, and identifying oneself as an AA member.

Effectiveness of MAAEZ

So, does MAAEZ work? Kaskutas and her colleagues at the School of Public Health at the University of California–Berkeley devised a study to find out. Working with two treatment centers, one in Northern California and one in Southern California, the researchers recruited 508 men and women (roughly two-thirds of them men) to participate in what researchers call an *on/off study*. These men and women were randomly assigned to one of two treatment programs. The first six sessions in both programs were identical with respect to content. This was the standard treatment and included topics that can be found in typical substance abuse treatment programs—addiction education, stress management and anger management, family education, and relapse prevention—all in the context of group discussions with a therapist. Also included was the standard recommendation to attend AA or NA meetings.

In the standard treatment condition (or "off condition"), these topics continued to be the focus of therapy for all of the following sessions. In contrast, the second group received the MAAEZ treatment, as described above, for the next six therapy sessions. This was labeled the "on condition." Then, after the six MAAEZ sessions, the "on" group returned to the standard treatment format.

If we were to draw a picture of this study, it would look like this:

OFF (Standard) - ➤ OFF (Standard)

OFF (Standard) - - - - - - ➤ ON (MAAEZ) - - - - - - ➤ OFF (Standard)

The entire group of 508 men and women were assessed periodically for alcohol and drug use, through both self-reports and urinalysis.

The researchers found that the "on" phase of treatment—the participants who attended the MAAEZ sessions—was associated with significantly higher rates of past-thirty-day abstinence from both alcohol and other drugs. After twelve months, 87.5 percent of participants in the group that had received MAAEZ were abstinent from alcohol and drugs as compared to 72.6 percent in the group that had remained in standard treatment. The standard treatment, then, was effective, but treatment that included MAAEZ was more effective.

The magnitude of the difference between the MAAEZ versus standard treatments in this study was similar to that found by Christine Timko and her associates in the study involving intensive referral to AA that we looked at earlier. The corresponding findings from two independent studies lend strength to the idea that making Twelve Step involvement a core part (in other words, the goal) of treatment increases that treatment's effectiveness.

Twelve Step Facilitation (TSF)

Twelve Step Facilitation, or TSF, like MAAEZ, seeks to bring the Twelve Step program front and center in treatment. I should point out that I am the principal author of the Twelve Step Facilitation protocols, which I initially developed in collaboration with several colleagues and have since developed several variants of—for example, for use with individuals who have both a substance use disorder and a mental illness. And while I have served as a collaborator and adviser in many of these studies, I have not played a role in data collection or analysis. In short, the findings reported here speak for themselves, not for me.

The stated goal of TSF is to facilitate the patient's active involvement in one or more Twelve Step fellowships. It seeks to do so through a combination of coaching and working through resistance. The "coaching" aspect of TSF includes educating the patient about basic AA concepts and "rules of the road," and suggesting and following up on specific ways of enhancing the person's involvement, such as sharing phone numbers or email addresses with other AA members.

The "working through resistance" aspect of TSF is accomplished by engaging the client in a dialogue about AA's concepts, helping identify appropriate meetings, talking about any reservations the patient may have about getting active in AA, correcting inaccurate stereotypes, managing expectations, and processing any negative experiences associated with Twelve Step fellowships. TSF can be delivered individually or, like MAAEZ, in a group format.

TSF is divided into a series of components or subprograms,

starting with a Core Program, which is administered to every TSF client. It consists of the following topics:

- *Assessment:* Briefly evaluates the severity of a substance use disorder as well as a history of prior attempts to deal with it

- *Acceptance:* Explores the patient's willingness to accept a diagnosis of alcohol use disorder as well as to accept abstinence as a goal

- *Surrender:* Explores the issue of reaching out to others as opposed to relying on personal willpower alone to overcome a substance use disorder

- *Getting active:* Coaches the patient on how to move from simple meeting attendance to active involvement in a Twelve Step fellowship

Taken as a whole, the TSF core program essentially consists of an in-depth client-therapist dialogue about the first three Steps of the Twelve Step program, followed by an effort at coaching the patient in how to get active by building a support network (via telephone, email, or texting), seeking out a sponsor, settling on a home meeting, and so on. (AA's Twelve Steps are listed at the back of this book.)

The desired end result of "getting active" is for the patient to identify himself or herself as a "member" of a Twelve Step fellowship. In that sense this fourth core topic aims to facilitate behavioral change, whereas the second and third topics work more on a cognitive level (accepting the idea that drinking or drug use has made a person's life "unmanageable," along with the idea that reaching out to others for help is the best solution).

TSF also offers an Elective Program, which consists of a set of topics that the therapist is free to choose from when working with an individual or group. Here are the topics in this Elective Program:

- *Genograms:* Traces alcohol or drug abuse (and consequences) through the client's family history using a "family tree" approach

- *Enabling:* Explores the issue of how loved ones can inadvertently "enable" alcohol or drug use, as well as how the substance user may encourage this

- *People, places, and routines:* Works with the patient to develop a "Lifestyle Contract" toward the goal of gradually replacing a lifestyle that supports alcohol or drug use with one that supports recovery

- *Emotions:* Helps the patient identify emotions, such as anger, social anxiety, boredom, or loneliness, that can trigger urges to drink or use

- *Moral inventories:* Helps the patient identify harmful consequences to self and others that may have resulted from alcohol or drug use

- *Relationships:* Introduces the idea that chronic alcohol and drug use disorders do harm to relationships, as well as advice on starting the healing process in recovery

Again, therapists choose those topics that seem most relevant to the particular client or group. In clinical trials, the topics of enabling; people, places, and routines; and emotions were most commonly chosen.

Finally, TSF includes a DVD, *Introduction to Twelve Step Groups,* designed to anticipate and correct any false stereotypes or expectations an individual might harbor about Twelve Step fellowships. The video features a diverse group of AA and NA members talking about their experiences. A narrator organizes this discussion into a series of topics, such as what to expect when going to a first Twelve Step meeting, what a sponsor is, and how AA is not a religion. In a way, this DVD seeks to accomplish what the use of an AA volunteer did in Timko's study of intensive referral to a Twelve Step fellowship.

Both MAAEZ and TSF sessions are highly structured and manual guided. They begin with a review of the client's "recovery life" in the time between sessions, proceed to a discussion of a specific topic, and end with a homework assignment to be completed between sessions. Indeed, they go well beyond generic interventions that begin and end at recommending AA attendance.

Effectiveness of TSF

TSF was first tested in the research project I mentioned in the beginning of this book, Project MATCH. This ambitious long-term study set out to determine not only whether three treatments for alcohol use disorders were effective, but also whether one treatment worked best for certain kinds of patients or problem severity. There were, accordingly, a large number of "matching" hypotheses about which treatments would work best for whom.

TSF was one of the three treatments, the others being cognitive behavioral therapy (CBT) and motivational enhancement therapy (MET). TSF is described above. CBT is a skills-based approach based on the assumption that drinking is a means of coping and that teaching people alternative coping skills, as well as other skills such as how to say no when offered a drink, will resolve the problem. CBT is well-established as a psychotherapeutic model and has been used to address issues ranging from depression to anxiety, as well as drinking. The researchers who developed CBT for use in MATCH described it this way:

CBT aims at training the patient to use active behavioral or cognitive coping methods to deal with
problems rather than relying on alcohol as a mal-
adaptive coping strategy.

CBT is also a manual-guided therapy. Topics that therapists
using CBT have to choose from include the following:

- coping with cravings and urges to drink
- managing thoughts about alcohol and drinking
- problem solving
- drink refusal skills
- planning for emergencies and coping with a lapse
- seemingly irrelevant decisions

The above are largely self-explanatory. In a session on drink
refusal skills, for example, the therapist coaches the client in
how to turn down offers to drink—how to say "no"—using role
playing if necessary. Seemingly irrelevant decisions can include
things like deciding to keep some liquor in the house "for drinking friends who might stop by." Such a decision can obviously increase the risk of a lapse. And planning for emergencies involves
creating stressful scenarios and then thinking about ways to cope
with them without drinking.

MET is a novel approach to recovery based on the notion that
people will do something about their drinking once they decide
it is a problem. Its developers describe it this way:

MET does not attempt to guide and train the client,
step by step, through recovery, but instead employs
motivational strategies to mobilize the client's own
change resources.

MET assumes that each individual will find his or her own solution at that point. What MET seeks to accomplish, through its own particular approach to counseling, is to move patients from a point where they do not see drinking as a problem (despite objective evidence to the contrary) to a point where they first recognize drinking as a problem and then decide to do something about it.

MET is what is known among professionals as a *process therapy*, meaning that it establishes rules that guide the interaction (the process) between the client and the therapist. Therapists learn and practice the following skills, which taken together are aimed at moving clients toward a decision to change their drinking behavior:

- *Expressing empathy:* Learning to "reflect" what the patient says in a way that communicates understanding on the part of the therapist. Example: "So you're saying that stress at your workplace is sky-high and that's why you now drink several beers after leaving work."

- *Developing discrepancy:* Pointing out (in a nonconfrontational manner) discrepancies between what the patient says and his or her actual behavior. Example: "I hear you saying that you don't really think drinking is a problem for you, but you did get that DUI and your doctor says you may be on the verge of being diagnosed with diabetes."

- *Rolling with resistance:* Not directly challenging or arguing with the patient—for instance, in reaction to positive results from a blood alcohol level test—but instead, when faced with strong resistance, falling back on expressing empathy. Example: "Okay, so you don't really think you have a problem or need to change your drinking behavior at this time."

- *Supporting self-efficacy:* Reinforcing any and all verbal expressions of confidence from the client about changing his or her drinking behavior. Example: "So you really think you can reduce your drinking if you set your mind to it."

Since Project MATCH, these three evidence-based approaches have been often practiced together in integrated treatment programs that emphasize an individualized approach, or combination of approaches, for helping each client at any given time in the treatment process.

Project MATCH Results

A total of 1,726 men and women (roughly three-fourths male) who had been diagnosed with alcohol use disorders (not just alcohol dependence) were randomly assigned to one of the three treatments: CBT, MET, or TSF. Of this group, almost 1,000 had not received prior treatment; the remainder were recruited as they completed alcohol treatment programs.

The outcomes that the Project MATCH researchers focused on were the two described earlier: how often participants abstained from drinking versus drinking (percent days abstinent, or PDA) and how much they drank when they did drink (drinks per drinking day, or DDD). These are the most commonly accepted recovery measures used by researchers, and they make intuitive sense.

The men and women treated through Project MATCH were followed for three years and assessed periodically using these measures. The data were analyzed separately for the participants who had never received treatment (the "outpatient" group) and those who received additional treatment after finishing an intensive treatment program (the "aftercare" group). This was done to help determine whether any of the three MATCH treatments worked better for one group versus the other.

Project MATCH was a researcher's dream in terms of the sheer amount and variety of information that was collected (and is still being analyzed) in different ways. The project, which spanned seven years, initially yielded two major publications, one summarizing its outcomes for individuals twelve months after they completed treatment and a second one that presented information on how the MATCH participants were doing three years after completing treatment. Let's look at each of these.

One-Year Post-Treatment Outcomes

Participants in the outpatient arm, who had not received prior treatment, reported abstaining from alcohol about three in every ten days (30 percent PDA) before entering treatment. After completing treatment, PDA had increased to between 80 and 90 percent for all three treatments (TSF, CBT, and MET). However, those who received TSF reported the highest percentage of days when they did not drink. A year later, the percentage of days when these men and women did not drink had decreased slightly but still hovered at the 80 percent mark, again with those who received TSF having a slight advantage.

As for how much they drank on those days when they did drink, the study participants in the outpatient arm reported drinking an average of eleven to thirteen drinks—in other words, a lot—prior to treatment. After they completed treatment, their DDD number decreased to two or three drinks on those occasions when they did drink, with the number of drinks per drinking day being the lowest for participants who underwent TSF as opposed to either the CBT or MET treatments.

Turning to the aftercare group, who entered Project MATCH after completing intensive treatment, they reported being abstinent only about 25 percent of the time just prior to entering Project MATCH and receiving one of its three treatments. This represents fewer sober days than those who had no prior treatment. It most likely reflects the reality that those in the aftercare group had more severe drinking problems than those in the outpatient group.

Following treatment, the percentage of days abstinent for this aftercare group was close to 95 percent, and a year later it was around 90 percent. With respect for how much they drank when they did drink, the aftercare group reported a staggering fifteen to twenty drinks per drinking day before treatment, which supports the idea that their problems on average were more severe than those in the outpatient arm. After they completed treatment, the drinks per drinking day among those in the aftercare group had decreased to about two drinks—a figure that was sustained a full year later.

Surprising Results

Some people—both researchers and clinicians—were surprised by the results from Project MATCH as reported in its one-year follow-up. This includes people who had been cynical about *all* treatments for alcohol use disorders, and who had expected much higher relapse rates than were found a year out. Then there were those who were clearly cheering for one treatment over the others, or were convinced that the Twelve Step approach was either "unproven" at best or a "cult" at worst. The finding that all three MATCH treatments (CBT, MET, and TSF) led to significant and sustained increases in abstinence rates and reductions in drinks per drinking day challenged these individuals' biases.

Other surprises lurked within the MATCH results. In particular, few of the "matching hypotheses" panned out. For example, TSF was not more effective for men than women, as predicted; nor was it less effective for those men and women whose diagnoses fell short of alcohol dependence. In effect, TSF was not just for men or just for those who had hit bottom.

The authors of this initial outcome publication (the Project MATCH Research Group) make one other point that is worth noting, especially in light of the research we've looked at up until now. They point out that AA attendance was not controlled in Project MATCH. In other words, whereas TSF deliberately encouraged AA attendance and sought to facilitate AA involvement, participants who were assigned to CBT and MET were also free to attend AA—and many did just that, particularly those who had completed prior treatment.

So one could argue that a true test of the effectiveness of TSF versus the other two MATCH treatments would require that the men and women assigned to CBT and MET refrain from attending AA meetings. But that would not really be feasible—and perhaps not ethical. And so we will never know if the advantage of TSF would have been greater had AA attendance been forbidden in the other treatments.

Three-Year Project MATCH Outcomes

The Project MATCH Research Group later reported on the drinking outcomes of the 952 men and women who had undergone treatment through the outpatient arm: those who had not received treatment prior to enrolling in MATCH. They found, first, that fully 30 percent of this group continued to be totally abstinent three years after treatment. Those who were not totally abstinent reported being abstinent two-thirds of the time. Finally, as was the case in the one-year follow-up, participants who received TSF showed an advantage of about 10 percent over those who received one of the other two treatments. If you recall in our review of MAAEZ, the men and women who received that intervention as part of their overall treatment also fared better than those who received only the standard treatment.

The one matching hypothesis that was supported three years following treatment concerned anger: men and women who scored higher on a scale measuring their tendency to get angry did better when they were assigned to motivational enhancement therapy. This hypothesis was originally made because MET is a highly nonconfrontational approach to treatment, so it seemed logical that people who are prone to anger might be turned off by even minor confrontations. While neither CBT nor TSF could be characterized as highly confrontational, therapists using them are certainly more likely to be challenging now and then than those who are using the MET approach. For patients who present as having a "short fuse," therapists who wish to pursue a therapy like TSF are wise to also use a reinforcing approach and to avoid challenging such clients, for example by questioning them a lot if they fail to attend any meetings in between therapy sessions.

As at the end of year one, at the three-year mark those who had received TSF treatment were attending more AA meetings than those who received CBT or MET. However, study participants who received CBT and MET still did go to some AA meetings. When looking at the effect of AA attendance on abstinence and drinks per drinking day, analysis revealed that going to AA meetings was a "causal factor"—that is, AA attendance was making a difference, contributing to both abstinence and reduced drinking, in *all three* treatments.

Network Support for Drinking

One of the most significant findings that emerged from the three-year follow-up of MATCH participants had to do with something called "network support for drinking." This refers to how much the individual's closest associates (friends and family) are people who drink and who therefore could be said to support drinking.

In contrast are friends and family who either don't drink or drink very little, and are therefore said to support sobriety as opposed to drinking.

Twelve Step fellowships like AA and NA (as well as other groups, such as Women for Sobriety and SMART Recovery) are built-in social networks that support sobriety as opposed to drinking. Project MATCH found that participants whose social networks tended to support drinking did better when the treatment they received was TSF as opposed to CBT or MET. Even three years after finishing treatment, the TSF group reported a higher percentage of days abstinent plus fewer drinks when they did drink as compared to those who received either the CBT or MET treatments.

These two outcome studies led one of the Project MATCH principal investigators to the following conclusion:

> On at least one time-honored outcome measure— the percentage of patients maintaining complete abstinence—those in the Twelve Step Facilitation

treatment fared significantly better at all follow-up points than did patients in the other two conditions—a substantial advantage of about 10 percentage points that endured across three years.

So far, then, both of the focused therapies we've looked at (MAAEZ and TSF), which have been evaluated through controlled clinical trials, support the view that actively promoting involvement in Twelve Step fellowships is effective for men and women with alcohol use disorders.

Replication

Researchers place a high value on *replication,* or repeated similar results. For example, if an independent researcher achieves the same or very similar positive results when using the same intervention in another place, at another time, and with a new group of participants, that finding lends credence to the idea that the intervention really works. In other words, replication is a safeguard of sorts against what might turn out to be a fluke—a one-off result.

Replication is so highly prized that it is one hurdle a therapeutic intervention needs to straddle in order to be considered "evidence-based," which qualifies it for inclusion in the National Registry of Evidence-based Programs and Practices (NREPP). The NREPP is overseen by the U.S. Department of Health and Human Services. As clinical practice in medicine and mental health moves more and more toward using evidence-based treatments, inclusion in an objective peer-reviewed source like the NREPP will become increasingly important, both to consumers who may want confirmation that a proposed treatment is effective and to the third-party payers (insurers) who pay for that treatment.

Kimberly Walitzer, PhD, is senior research director at the Research Institute on Addictions (RIA), which is part of the State University of New York–Buffalo. In 1993 the National Institute on Alcohol Abuse and Alcoholism (NIAAA) designated the RIA as a National Alcohol Research Center.

In 2009, Walitzer and her RIA colleagues reported the results of a clinical trial involving 169 individuals (including 57 women) diagnosed as alcohol dependent (alcoholic) who were randomly assigned to one of three treatments:

- *Treatment as usual (TAU):* TAU is a twelve-session treatment that focuses on such issues as problem-solving skills, drink refusal skills, and relaxation.

- *Twelve Step Facilitation (TSF):* As described above, TSF seeks to facilitate active involvement in AA through education and coaching.

- *Motivational enhancement therapy (MET):* Also described above, MET seeks to help clients move from a position in which they do not believe they have a drinking problem to the point of deciding that a problem exists and needs to be addressed. MET does not, however, advocate for one particular "solution" to the problem, such as the Twelve Step AA program.

This study essentially stands as a replication of what was found in Project MATCH. Here is what Walitzer learned:

> Participants in the TSF condition reported more AA meeting attendance, more evidence of active involvement in AA and a higher percentage of days

abstinent relative to participants in the treatment-as-usual group. The motivational enhancement approach to facilitating AA had no effect on outcome measures.

In this study, AA "involvement" again meant things like having a sponsor, identifying oneself as an AA member, working the AA Steps, and celebrating AA sobriety anniversaries.

Summing Up

The RIA study stands as a replication of Project MATCH. It also presents further evidence supporting the effectiveness of treatments such as TSF and MAAEZ, which bring the Twelve Step program into the spotlight of treatment. Rather than using AA as an adjunct to treatment, the Twelve Step program is the focus of treatment for these interventions.

So far we have looked at AA's Twelve Step program and its effectiveness from a variety of perspectives, beginning with what AA members themselves say through AA's periodic membership surveys. Then we looked at research on AA attendance and involvement to see what it could tell us about AA and its relationship to recovery. From there we moved into examining treatments that not only monitored AA attendance but actively encouraged it. And finally we looked at two therapies that bring the Twelve Step program front and center in treatment, aiming to educate and coach patients to attend AA and get active in its program. The results at this point seem unequivocal:

- Getting into some form of counseling and starting AA at the same time is a winning combination if you want to stay sober.

- Getting involved in the AA Twelve Step fellowship leads to superior results than simply attending meetings.

- Identifying yourself as an AA member makes a positive difference.

- Therapy that actively facilitates AA involvement is superior to treatment that does not include this focus.

In the next chapter, we will look at an issue that continues to be controversial: so-called controlled or nonproblem drinking as a goal, as opposed to abstinence. Let's see what light research can shed on that.

Food for Thought

1. Do you feel you've learned enough about how Twelve Step peer recovery works to make good decisions about attending meetings and how to use them? How can you fill in any gaps in your understanding of peer support groups and the Steps?

2. Which of the following factors do you think are most important for your recovery program, and what can you do to achieve them?

   a. understanding your family history

   b. dealing with the enabling behaviors of loved ones

   c. living a recovery lifestyle

   d. understanding and dealing with emotions

   e. doing a moral inventory to address short-comings and identify strengths

   f. healing relationships

3. Does learning about the effectiveness of the Twelve Step recovery program in studies such as Project MATCH increase your belief that it might work for you if you follow the guidelines for success? What might help overcome any remaining doubts?

◆

The Great Abstinence Debate

In chapter 1 it was noted that according to AA's own estimates, roughly half of people who try Alcoholics Anonymous stop attending meetings within three months. AA knows little about these individuals—their drinking habits, their motivations for going to AA in the first place, or their reasons for stopping—because AA simply does not conduct that kind of research. The general dropout rate was reported in a paper written for AA, "Comments on AA's Triennial Surveys," whose authors commented that AA had a tradition of welcoming newcomers and that perhaps it should consider emphasizing that tradition even more moving forward.

Regardless of this recommendation, it is clear that not everyone who tries the AA Twelve Step program stays with it. On the other hand, we have reviewed a significant body of research that supports the efficacy of Twelve Step programs for those who choose to pursue and get involved in fellowships like AA, NA, or Women for Sobriety.

Another finding at the root of the controversy that we'll discuss in this chapter is this: some individuals who choose to participate in the AA Twelve Step program end up being what is called "nonproblem" drinkers; that is, while they may not be problem-free, they drink at a level that does not result in severe negative consequences. This raises the question of exactly where we should draw the line between "problem" versus "nonproblem" drinking.

Until recently, it was generally accepted that there are roughly three categories of drinkers: first the "nonproblem" or "low-risk" drinkers, most of whom drink alcohol socially and don't routinely drink to intoxication, and then two categories of "problem" drinkers—people who abuse alcohol and people who are alcohol dependent. The recommended treatment and recovery plan for either diagnosis of problem drinking included Twelve Step group attendance and required total abstinence—especially for those who were alcohol dependent.

In 2013, the American Psychiatric Association published new diagnostic classifications for substance users, including drinkers (more about these classifications later in this chapter) that have opened the door for re-evaluation of, and some controversy about, when a person is a problem drinker versus a nonproblem or low-risk drinker—and when the person is at a low enough risk that abstinence isn't required.

Defining Low-Risk Drinking

As it turns out, there has also been some research, as well as official advisories, on the subject of just what constitutes low-risk (nonproblem) drinking. A study conducted by Martha Sanchez-Craig and colleagues at the Addiction Research Foundation in Toronto and published in the *American Journal of Public Health*, looked at 235 clients (91 women, 144 men) who participated in three separate but related studies.

These men and women had all signed up for programs that

advertised educational materials for people who wanted "to quit or cut down" on their drinking. Note that by including the words *cut down* these ads opened the door to options other than abstinence, including voluntarily reducing drinking based on education or a single-session counseling or education program. Collectively such efforts are referred to as "secondary prevention" programs because they are targeted at people whose drinking has not (at least not yet) led to serious consequences.

At the outset, and again twelve months later, these individuals were asked if their drinking had caused any problems in the following areas of their lives: health, relationships, aggression, work, finances, and the law. Those who reported severe problems in any of these areas were weeded out at the beginning, so that the remainder of the study included only men and women who initially reported drinking-related problems that were mild at worst and did not require more intensive intervention.

The researchers were interested in seeing how much and how often these individuals—who at the outset said they wanted to change their drinking behavior—drank over the course of a year, and what if any new consequences they experienced after receiving these secondary prevention materials. That information in turn would help them to establish cutoffs that separated problem drinking from nonproblem drinking.

After one year, the group was divided into two categories based on both their reported drinking-related problems and their alcohol consumption:

- *Problem-free drinking:* No reported drinking-related problems
- *Problem drinking:* At least one reported problem in one of the above areas

Here are the cutoff points between problem-free and problem drinking that these researchers found, which turned out to be different for men and women:

- *Men:* No more than four drinks on any given day and no more than sixteen drinks per week
- *Women:* No more than three drinks on any given day and no more than twelve drinks per week

The above "lines" were what separated problem from non-problem drinkers in this study. The National institute on Alcohol Abuse and Alcoholism (NIAAA) also publishes a booklet titled *Rethinking Drinking* that recommends similar limits for low-risk drinking. Those limits are, for men, no more than four drinks on any given day and no more than fourteen drinks per week; for women, no more than three drinks per day and no more than seven drinks per week.

Readers can decide for themselves which of the above cutoffs make the most sense to them. However, it's important to remember that the lower cutoffs for women are not based on the fact that men on average weigh more than women. This is a common assumption, but it is wrong. Women actually metabolize alcohol more slowly than men do. The result is that the blood alcohol level in a woman's body will be higher than in a man's even if they consume the same number of drinks. Beyond that, women's livers produce less of the enzyme that neutralizes the chemical acetaldehyde, which is a by-product of alcohol and is classified as a carcinogen. Because women metabolize alcohol more slowly than men do, there is consequently more of this carcinogen in their bodies for a longer time after they drink.

To add another wrinkle to this discussion, it turns out that it is easier for our bodies to metabolize alcohol when we consume it in small doses. That means that having one glass of wine a night for a woman (seven drinks per week) is safer than drinking three glasses on one night and four on another. The same is true for men: seven drinks in two days may equal fourteen drinks a week, but such consumption is more risky than having two drinks a day for seven days.

A Questionable Premise?

The finding that some men and women who go to AA end up being nonproblem drinkers has led some people to propose the following: if some AA members are actually nonproblem drinkers, why won't AA set "controlled drinking," as opposed to abstinence, as a goal from the outset? Let's take a look at what research has to tell us about this premise.

The idea of controlled or moderate drinking as a goal is probably most closely associated with the organization Moderation Management (MM). MM was established by Audrey Kishline in 1994 and seeks to be an alternative to AA for men and women who do not wish to stop drinking, but rather to moderate their drinking and thereby reduce its detrimental consequences.

So, what do we know about MM? Some answers can be found in research conducted by Keith Humphreys, PhD. Humphreys is professor of psychiatry and behavioral sciences at the Stanford University Medical School. He is also honorary professor of psychiatry at the Institute of Psychiatry at Maudsley Hospital, King's College London.

Humphreys and his research team compared self-identified members of MM with self-identified members of AA. They looked at demographics—who attends AA versus MM—as well as the relative severity of the drinking problems in the two groups.

What this group found, first, was that the drinking problems among those who preferred MM was significantly less severe than that of AA members. In effect, men and women drawn to MM had "self-selected" the program based on the mild to moderate negative consequences they had experienced related to their drinking. So the two programs—MM and AA—appeal to two different groups of people.

Additionally, members of MM were more likely to be female, younger than thirty-five years old, and currently employed. Those demographics cast MM membership in pretty stark contrast to AA membership (consider, for example, the AA member surveys we reviewed earlier with respect to age, plus with the severity of drinking problems reported by the men and women typically recruited for the research we've been reviewing).

Humphreys also found that the MM group as a whole was high on every social and demographic factor associated with being able to reduce drinking: being more highly educated, having full-time jobs, having family support, and so on. In effect, the MM members had the advantage of a social network that did not support heavy drinking, but would support their decision to drink at a moderate level. Based on these factors the MM members had the most favorable prognosis for succeeding at moderation. But keep in mind: as a group they are very different from those who choose AA and abstinence over moderation.

One interesting finding from the Humphreys study is that about 15 percent of MM members reported experiencing three or more of the following symptoms at least once in the six months before they started attending MM: tremors (shaking when not intoxicated), delirium tremens, blackouts while drinking, convulsions after drinking, craving for a drink on waking up in the morning, and problems with their families or jobs as a result of drinking. These of course are all symptoms of a severe drinking problem, not a moderate one. Yet only 3 percent of these heavy drinkers decided to pursue abstinence as opposed to controlled drinking as their personal goal through MM. There is no way of knowing how many of these individuals went on to suffer more severe consequences from their drinking or who may eventually have elected to pursue abstinence. We do know from her memoir, however, that Audrey Kishline herself eventually concluded that abstinence was her best option. Sadly, this came after she was convicted of killing two people while driving drunk.

In his conclusion, Humphreys stated that the vast majority of MM members (85 percent) have low-severity drinking problems and enjoy lifestyles that are conducive to reducing their drinking in lieu of stopping. At the same time, the other 15 percent are worrisome, leading these researchers to conclude that it would be unrealistic to recommend MM to all individuals who are experiencing problems related to drinking. With that provision, moderation may be an acceptable goal for younger people who have stable lifestyles, who have social networks that do not support heavy drinking, and who have none of the signs of alcohol dependence cited above. In that case MM may be a useful source of support.

Self-Control Training

William R. Miller is emeritus distinguished professor of psychology and psychiatry at the University of New Mexico, where he was also director of the Center on Alcoholism, Substance Abuse, and Addictions. Miller is the principal author of motivational enhancement therapy, which was discussed in the previous chapter. Miller is a multitalented man who, in addition to being a renowned researcher on addictions, has an interest in the phenomenon of *quantum change,* or how people can experience epiphanies that alter the course of their lives. In retirement he continues to serve as a consultant to substance abuse researchers as well as writes poetry and composes chorale music.

Miller was interested in studying the effectiveness of a treatment program whose goal would not be abstinence from alcohol, but rather moderation in drinking. So he set out, in collaboration with Ricardo Munoz of the University of California–San Francisco, to create and evaluate a treatment for drinking problems that they labeled behavioral self-control (BSC). This treatment—much like TSF and MAAEZ described earlier—is manual guided, is delivered by trained professionals, and consists of a series of modules:

- *Goal-setting:* Determining the client's goal for how much he or she drinks

- *Self-monitoring:* Keeping a log of how much the client drinks each day

- *Self-reinforcement:* Learning ways to reinforce meeting drinking goals

- *Identifying high-risk situations:* Determining what the client should avoid

- *Alternatives to drinking:* Exploring other ways of dealing with stress—for example, with anxiety or anger—besides drinking

Miller and his colleagues studied four groups whose drinking problems varied in intensity. These groups were evaluated at three, five, seven, and eight years after completing behavioral self-control training. Of the 140 individuals (45 percent of them women) who began the study, 94 were able to be followed and 16 refused to participate in the follow-ups. The authors note that the status of those who dropped out could not be known. This of course is by now familiar to us: we cannot know the fate of those men and women who stop going to AA or who drop out of treatment. The authors do conjecture that these dropouts may not have fared as well, but as reasonable as that hypothesis sounds it's still just a guess.

Let's look at what happened to the 94 who were evaluated eight years after they completed BSC. Here is what the researchers led by Miller found:

- 23 reported abstaining altogether from alcohol by choice (24 percent).

- 14 reported being able to control their drinking without significant consequences (15 percent).

- 22 had reduced their drinking but were considered still impaired as a consequence of drinking (23 percent).

- 35 still had significant drinking problems and were classified as "unremitted" (37 percent).

So what can we conclude about this effort at controlled drinking? First, it appears that a small minority of problem drinkers (15 percent) were able to reduce their drinking to a point where it was not causing a significant disruption in their lives. Does that mean that BSC doesn't work very well? No, though it suggests that the BSC program can work for roughly fifteen out of one hundred problem drinkers. For the majority, though (57 of 94, or 61 percent), a decision to try to moderate their drinking left them either still impaired or no better off eight years later. Meanwhile, almost a quarter eventually decided on abstinence as their goal.

A footnote at the end of this study is intriguing. The authors comment that, in their interviews with the men and women

who failed to improve through the behavioral self-control training, that failure was still not enough to motivate them to change
their drinking goals and, in particular, to set abstinence as a goal.
Some people, it seems, will continue to struggle and stumble for
a long time rather than change direction—not unlike many of
the stories one hears at AA meetings!

The best that can be said for both BSC and MM is that they
appear to work for some people, but that by no means are they
a viable alternative to abstinence for everyone with a drinking
problem.

The Goal Makes a Difference

The finding that even an experience of failure at controlled
drinking is not enough to convince some people that they should
consider abstinence as an alternate goal leads to this interesting
question: Does an individual's goal make a difference? Specifically, can one's goal predict recovery?

As it turns out this is yet another question on which objective
research has a lot to teach us. Let's look at a series of studies in
which researchers assessed clients' stated goals and then followed
them to see how those goals affected their recovery, as well as
research in which therapists tried to influence those goals.

The first study we'll consider was conducted by researchers from the University of California–Los Angeles and Yale
University. The 1,226 participants in this study (798 men and
428 women) had all been diagnosed as alcohol dependent (in
other words, with a severe alcohol use disorder) and were part of a
larger study involving a combination of therapy plus medication.

These individuals were recruited from eleven U.S. cities. At
the outset each participant was asked to identify his or her goal
in seeking treatment from the following list:

- *Controlled drinking:* I want to use alcohol in a controlled manner—to be in control of how often I use and how much I use.

- *Complete abstinence:* I want to quit using alcohol once and for all, to be totally abstinent, and never use alcohol again for the rest of my life.

- *Conditional abstinence:* I want to be totally abstinent from all alcohol use for a period of time, after which I will make a new decision about whether I will use alcohol again in any way.

The treatment phase of this study lasted sixteen weeks and consisted of up to twenty individual sessions. An attempt was made to incorporate aspects from all three of the treatment approaches described earlier: cognitive behavioral therapy, Twelve Step Facilitation, and motivational enhancement therapy. The outcome of treatment was measured in ways we've also already discussed. They included percent days abstinent (PDA) and drinks per drinking day (DDD). In addition the researchers looked at how long it might take someone to relapse to heavy drinking, calling it days to relapse (DTR).

This was another large, national study, similar to Project MATCH, which we reviewed in chapter 3. With multisite studies, the results are much less likely to be influenced by the particular form of treatment that may be favored by researchers at one particular university or treatment center. One could say that in multi-site studies such biases tend to "come out in the wash," while more robust results emerge.

So what did this study teach us about the role that a person's goal might play in his or her recovery? Here is what the authors wrote in their discussion of their findings:

It was hypothesized that patients whose drinking goals were oriented toward complete abstinence would have better treatment outcomes as measured by a greater percentage of days abstinent, longer period until relapse, and an overall better clinical outcome. These hypotheses were supported by the present study.

More specifically, the men and women who chose abstinence as their goal had the best outcome after treatment. Those with a goal of "controlled drinking" had the worst drinking outcomes. Finally, those who selected "conditional abstinence," as defined above, had outcomes in between the two other groups.

The findings of this study suggest that a person's goal for seeking treatment or even just for doing something about a drinking problem does indeed make a difference, with a goal of abstaining being associated with the best long-term outcomes as measured by drinking versus not drinking and length of sobriety. Deciding to abstain for some period of time and then re-evaluate one's goal appears to lead to some sort of middle-ground outcome. We could conjecture that conditional abstinence as a goal reflects ambivalence—a cognitive waypoint between controlled drinking and abstinence.

Let's turn now to a study conducted by Sharon Hall, PhD, and her colleagues at the University of California–San Francisco and San Francisco General Hospital. Hall holds the position of professor of psychiatry and is also the leader of the Tobacco Control Program of the Helen Diller Family Comprehensive Cancer Center. She and her colleagues investigate treatments for addiction to opiates and tobacco as well as alcohol. As long ago as

1990 they reported the results of a study related to how goals affect treatment effectiveness.

This research team followed 225 individuals who had sought treatment for problems related to smoking (68 people), alcohol (85 people), or opiate use (72 people). They all had completed treatment programs that emphasized abstinence—from cigarettes, alcohol, or opiates—as opposed to controlled use or moderation. They then assessed this group for several things:

- *Commitment to abstinence:* Participants were asked to rate their "desire to quit" on a scale from 0 to 10, with 10 being the highest. They were also asked to endorse one of the following goals: total abstinence, abstinence but realizing that slips were possible, occasional use when an urge to use is strong, temporary abstinence for a period of time, and controlled use.

- *Stressful life events:* Participants completed a scale that assessed just how stressful their lives might be, to see if there was any connection to relapsing to smoking, drinking, or opiate use.

- *Mood scale:* This was used to assess moods such as anger, depression, fear, and fatigue, again to determine if these moods might be related to relapse.

Here is how these researchers summarized their findings:

A major finding of our study was that return to substance use for clients in treatment for alcohol, opiate, and nicotine dependence is predicable from their abstinence goal. Subjects with the most restrictive goal, absolute abstinence, were less likely to slip and less likely to relapse after a slip than subjects with less demanding goals. This relation held independent of drug group.

In this study, those men and women who endorsed "conditional abstinence"—they were open to reassessing their goal at some point and were willing to allow for occasional slips—did *worse* than those who endorsed total abstinence. These findings take on added significance when we look at what Hall and her colleagues found regarding moods and stress, which was that these factors were *not* predictive of slips or relapse. In short, it was the goal that made the difference.

In their conclusions on the relationship between personal goals and recovery, the authors offer this cautionary advice:

> Our results suggest caution when encouraging clients
> to embrace goals other than absolute abstinence. They
> also cast doubt on the importance of negative moods
> and stress in causing relapse.

There are two more studies relevant to this issue of personal goals and how they relate to recovery. The first was conducted by a team of researchers from the Center for Alcohol and Addiction Studies at Brown University in Rhode Island and led by Molly Magill.

Magill received her doctorate in social work research from Boston University. Her colleague, Robert Stout, PhD, has been named a principal investigator on no less than forty-three research projects funded by the National Institute on Alcohol Abuse and Alcoholism, the National Institute of Mental Health, and the National Institute on Drug Abuse.

Stout and Magill were interested in how two different kinds of therapist behavior might influence how much a person in treatment for a drinking problem actually drinks. Observing therapist-patient interactions, they used measures that assessed two distinct kinds of interactions, as follows:

- *Commitment to change:* How much the therapist encouraged the patient to commit to changing his or her drinking behavior during therapy sessions

- *Ambivalence:* How much the therapist explored a patient's mixed feelings about changing his or her drinking behavior

When focusing on "commitment to change" in treatment, the therapist encourages the patient to say things to that effect—for instance by posing questions like, "On a scale of 1 to 10, with 10 meaning most committed, how committed are you today to changing your drinking behavior?"

The therapist also talks with the patient about steps he or she can take to make changes. For example, if the patient makes a comment like "I think I do have a drinking problem," the therapist will reinforce that thought and then go a step further, nodding and saying something like "It does look that way. So what do you think would be a good first step toward changing your drinking?"

In contrast, the therapist whose focus is on "ambivalence" will be accepting of statements like "I may have a drinking problem, but I'm not really sure," without attempting to move the patient toward actually acknowledging a problem or doing something about it. When working in this mode, the therapist never challenges the patient, for example by pointing out some serious negative consequences that have been the result of drinking.

Theoretically speaking, the two approaches described above are similar in that both are based on the notion that people change only when they decide they need to change. To change one's drinking behavior, a person must first move from not believing that there is a problem, to contemplating that there may be a problem, to deciding a problem does exist, and finally to deciding to do something about it. The difference between the therapeutic approaches of commitment and ambivalence is therefore one of style—which style of interaction will be more effective in moving the patient toward accepting a problem and acting to fix it?

Motivational enhancement therapy (MET), which was described in chapter 3, trains therapists to utilize both of the above strategies in therapy sessions with patients. Magill and Stout wanted to know how much each therapeutic style contributed to patients' staying sober. So they analyzed the therapist-patient interactions and then correlated these with how much the patients drank. Their subjects were drawn from two sources: outpatient programs and aftercare programs for people completing inpatient treatment.

Here is what the researchers learned:

> Therapist effort to elicit commitment to change alcohol use was associated with greater rates of abstinence among both outpatient and aftercare participants. However, therapist focus on ambivalence was associated with greater drinking among outpatient participants, and when motivation was low, among aftercare participants.

These findings led the research team to conclude that a therapeutic style focused on commitment is an "active ingredient" in treatment success while a focus on ambivalence, as defined above, is not as effective in promoting change.

Here again we have objective evidence supporting the gen-

eral notion that a person's goals for change are a powerful deter-
minant of that change. One could even argue that *goals are apt
to become self-fulfilling prophecies.* In particular, setting a goal of
abstinence and committing to it leads to better outcomes than
setting a goal for either controlled drinking (as opposed to abstinence) or conditional abstinence (the intention to abstain, but
just for a period of time).

The last study we will examine in this discussion was conducted
by researchers at Massachusetts General Hospital and Harvard
Medical School and led by John Kelly, PhD. Kelly is the program director of the Addiction Recovery Management Services
(ARMS) at Massachusetts General Hospital and associate professor of psychiatry at Harvard Medical School. In addition, Kelly
serves as a consultant to the White House Office of National
Drug Control Policy.

Kelly and his co-researcher, M. Claire Greene, chose the
intriguing title *Where There's a Will There's a Way* to report
their findings of a study involving 302 young adults (average
age twenty, 74 percent male) who underwent residential treatment for substance use disorders. These young men and women
struggled with alcohol and, to an almost equal degree, cannabis, followed by opiates and cocaine. This is important to note
because today, as compared to twenty or thirty years ago, polysubstance abuse is increasingly the norm, particularly among
younger people. It is now difficult, in fact, to find a large group
of men and women who use *only* alcohol. Twelve Step recovery
groups such as NA and CA are generally more accepting today
of people addicted to multiple substances. AA itself has evolved
to the point where many of its members feel more comfortable
acknowledging that they are addicted to other drugs besides

alcohol, although they are still encouraged to focus on their drinking in meetings. Abstinence for all Twelve Step recovery groups means not using any mood-altering substance, whether you consider yourself addicted to it or not.

These researchers were interested in exploring two factors that relate to the issue of goals and motivation that we've been looking at here. The first is called *self-efficacy,* the extent to which an individual is confident that he or she can achieve a goal. In a sense self-efficacy boils down to self-confidence, in this case with respect to staying clean and sober. It was measured by asking study participants to rate themselves on a scale of 1 (not confident) to 10 (very confident) on this question: *how confident are you that you will be able to stay clean and sober in the next ninety days?*

The second factor that Kelly was interested in is called *motivation for recovery.* It is measured by asking participants to rate themselves, on a scale of 1 (strongly disagree) to 6 (strongly agree) on a series of statements such as

- Staying sober is the most important thing in my life.
- I am totally committed to staying off alcohol/drugs.

Looking at these statements, it's clear that motivation for recovery means abstinence as opposed to controlled use, with higher scores indicating stronger commitment to abstinence.

Following this group of young adults after they completed treatment, the researchers found that both of the factors they measured related to outcome three, six, and again twelve months later. In other words, both self-efficacy and motivation predicted sustained recovery. However, they also found that the effect of one factor depended in part on the effect of the other. They described the relationship in this way:

- For those men and women who expressed *high* self-confidence that they could stay clean and sober, motivation for recovery increased their chances for sustained recovery, albeit modestly. High self-confidence about one's ability to stay clean and sober, in effect, can play at least a minor role in promoting recovery *if* one is also motivated to abstain from alcohol and drugs.

- For those men and women who were *less* self-confident about their ability to stay clean and sober, *motivation for recovery* improved their chances a great deal.

Once again, then, it appears that a person's goal is a major factor in recovery. These results also suggest, though, that self-confidence and commitment are not synonymous but represent two factors that can interact in ways that either help or hinder recovery. In an ideal scenario that offers the best chance of achieving one's goal, the person is highly motivated to stay clean and sober, *and* has self-confidence in his or her ability to do so.

If we were to step back and take in the body of research we've reviewed in this chapter, there is little doubt that a person's goals, and in particular a commitment to abstinence (as opposed to controlled drinking or even temporary abstinence) is consistently associated with better outcomes for men and women—young and old—who seek help for a significant drinking problem. That decision and its outcome are also poignantly described by authors who have chronicled their journeys from alcoholism to sobriety. These include books like Pete Hamill's *A Drinking Life* and Caroline Knapp's *Drinking: A Love Story*. Both of these people—like many others—were "high-functioning alcoholics" whose talent and motivation enabled them to be productive despite the progressive ravages of alcoholism. Eventually, however, the addiction and its consequences led them to make the decision to quit and to set abstinence as their goal. As Hamill describes it, he then discovered that "life without addiction is better."

So, does this end the great abstinence debate? Not necessarily. Rather than seeking to end the debate once and for all, it might be better for us to pause and rethink and redefine it.

Rethinking Abstinence and Controlled Drinking

There is no real room for doubt, based on the objective research we've been looking at, about the effectiveness of the AA Twelve Step program for helping men and women sustain recovery—at least for those who commit to following it. Time and again our review of carefully designed studies from major research centers has affirmed this. We also know from AA's membership surveys what activities are associated with recovery. We know from researchers who have followed men and women post-treatment that greater AA attendance predicts recovery. And, further, we know that setting a goal of abstinence and committing to that goal is vital to sustained recovery. Beyond that we have seen that therapies that "dig in" and seek to actively facilitate Twelve Step involvement are more effective than those that simply recommend AA, and that therapists who actively pursue commitment to change get better results than those who simply accept a patient's ambivalence. Finally, it is not merely attendance that appears to make the difference; rather, it is identifying oneself as a "member" of a Twelve Step fellowship—as being on the inside looking out, as opposed to being a mere outside observer.

So where does the idea of *moderation* fit in—if anywhere? Despite its effectiveness, AA continues to be criticized by those who see its Twelve Step program as rigid in promoting abstinence as the sole solution to an alcohol use disorder. Some go so far as to liken AA to the temperance movements of the nineteenth and twentieth centuries. We should ask ourselves: is there any merit to their position?

Temperance and AA

What is popularly known as the temperance movement first appeared on the European continent in the late eighteenth and early nineteenth centuries and then spread to the United States. It coincided with two social developments: the rise of "hard liquor" with a stronger alcohol content as a readily available source of alcohol; and subsequent increases in spousal and child abuse, predominantly by men, that are overwhelmingly attributed to heavy use of hard liquor.

Before distilling techniques emerged that could produce liquors of higher proof, it was common for people to drink beverages that contained alcohol such as hard cider partly because much drinking water was muddied or ill-tasting. In response to this practice, one part of the temperance movement involved constructing and maintaining "temperance fountains" that provided clean, cool potable water.

Many of those who identified with temperance (often women who had suffered personally from the epidemic of alcohol abuse) promoted a goal of abstinence. Even from the beginning, however, others within the temperance movement advocated for "levelness" or moderation rather than abstinence. That faction, however, appeared to lose ground over time to those—many from the evangelical movement—who sought to ban alcohol entirely from society.

The temperance movement scored its biggest victory—and that a pyrrhic one at best—in the United States with Prohibition, the eighteenth amendment to the Constitution, which lasted from

1919 to 1933. Prohibition became notorious for the problem it did not eradicate (alcohol abuse) and the ones it did create (bootlegging, organized crime). It's safe to say that Prohibition left behind a bad taste (no pun intended) in the collective conscious of many Americans. That negativity lingers to this day, in part in the form of the bias against AA and its Twelve Step program. I have heard more than once, for example, about how America and consequently AA are "hung up" on abstinence.

But is AA truly hung up on abstinence? Let's see what AA itself has to say about that in its "Big Book," *Alcoholics Anonymous*. First there is this, on page 20:

> Moderate drinkers have little trouble in giving up liquor entirely if they have good reason for it. They can take it or leave it alone.
>
> Then we have a certain type of hard drinker. He may have the habit badly enough to gradually impair him, physically and mentally. It may cause him to die a few years before his time. If a sufficiently strong reason—ill health, falling in love, change of environment, or the warning of a doctor—becomes operative, this man can also stop or moderate, although he may find it difficult and troublesome and may even need medical attention.

Later, on pages 108–109, we find this passage, addressed to the drinker's spouse:

> Your husband may be only a heavy drinker. His drinking may be constant or it may be heavy only on certain occasions. Perhaps he spends too much money for liquor. It may be slowing him up mentally and physically, but he does not see it. Sometimes he is a

source of embarrassment to you and his friends. He is positive he can handle his liquor, that it does him no harm, that drinking is necessary in his business. He would probably be insulted if he were called an alcoholic. This world is full of people like him. Some will moderate or stop altogether, and some will not. Of those who keep on, a good number will become true alcoholics after a while.

From its inception AA and its Twelve Step program of recovery was aimed not at people like the above, but at those who, despite their best efforts, had lost the ability to moderate their drinking. These were men and women for whom alcohol had made their lives "unmanageable," and who had tried (without success) to stop or limit their drinking many times.

Should we interpret the history of AA to mean that we should wait until we "crash and burn" to decide on abstinence as a goal? Not at all. I've personally met a number of people who had at some point come to see themselves as problem drinkers and decided not to moderate, but to quit drinking altogether. And they, like Pete Hamill, found that life, in many ways, was better for it.

Judging by the above excerpts, though, one has to conclude that AA itself never prescribed abstinence as the remedy for all drinkers, including "problem drinkers." Do these individuals experience negative consequences related to their drinking? Yes. But are they alcoholics? Not necessarily. Some may move on to become alcoholics, as the last excerpt suggests, but others may moderate their drinking. This is consistent with research we looked at earlier, which found that *some* men and women who underwent treatment for an alcohol use disorder, as well as *some* men and women who chose AA for a while, ended up being so-called moderate drinkers.

A Different Perspective

Rather than continue the debate about abstinence versus controlled drinking, it might be more productive to reconsider the way we as a society view drinking problems and how mental health professionals diagnose and treat them.

For many years, professionals relied on criteria developed by the American Psychiatric Association as a basis for diagnosis. Those criteria were published in its *Diagnostic and Statistical Manual of Mental Disorders,* 4th edition, or *DSM-IV.* It identified just the two categories of drinking problems discussed earlier that qualified for a formal diagnosis: alcohol abuse and alcohol dependence. To be officially diagnosed as alcohol dependent (alcoholism), an individual had to experience symptoms of withdrawal when he or she stopped drinking. These symptoms include sweating, tremors, diarrhea, and even seizures. In addition, the individual needed to show signs of tolerance, meaning that more liquor was required over time to become intoxicated. In severe cases, this tolerance eventually reverses itself—as liver function deteriorates, alcohol is not metabolized, so even small amounts can lead to intoxication.

The above symptoms of withdrawal and tolerance are severe, and a small proportion of men and women who have drinking problems will experience them. Nevertheless, these were the criteria often used to justify treatment, particularly residential or inpatient treatment.

The *DSM-IV* included a second class of alcohol use disorders, called alcohol abuse. To qualify for this alternative diagnosis, the individual still needed to experience rather severe signs and symptoms stemming from alcohol use. For example, the individual must have experienced the aftereffects of drinking while at work or school, and have neglected work, child care, or household responsibilities. The person may also have used alcohol in hazardous situations, such as driving, or had legal problems directly related to drinking.

In reality, the traditional diagnoses of alcohol abuse and alcohol dependence did not differ that much in this diagnostic schema. In fact, the sole symptom that significantly separated them was withdrawal. But what about those men and women who drink well beyond what is generally considered low-risk drinking, as discussed earlier, yet do not meet the criteria for a formal diagnosis? When we look at their drinking behavior, should we conclude that they are essentially problem-free?

In its newest revision of its *Diagnostic and Statistical Manual of Mental Disorders* (5th ed.; *DSM-5*), the APA dropped the above categorical schema of drinking problems in favor of a dimensional one. They replaced the two diagnostic categories of abuse and dependence with a schema that identifies alcohol use disorders as existing along a spectrum. This spectrum can be thought of as a continuum that runs from mild to moderate to severe depending on how many symptoms a person exhibits in relation to drinking.

While some have responded to the *DSM-5* by accusing the APA and its new diagnostic schema of trying to overdiagnose drinking problems, I would argue that it more accurately reflects the "drinking world" today. That drinking world can be represented graphically as follows:

The Drinking World

Alcoholic

Low Risk "Social" Drinking	Mild Problem Drinking	Moderate Problem Drinking	Severe Problem Drinking

© Harvard University 2012

At the extreme left of this spectrum is low-risk drinking as defined by the NIAAA. As that agency points out, however, low-risk is not synonymous with no-risk. Links between alcohol consumption and cancer have been established through research, and those researchers point out that there is no lower limit at which point the risk to health (including cancer) is zero. Additionally, as noted previously, having one glass of wine a night for seven nights is less risky (for a woman) than having three glasses on one night and four on another, even though both come out to seven glasses a week. The reason, again, is that a woman's liver is not as capable of metabolizing the chemical by-products of alcohol as quickly as a man's. One of those by-products is a known carcinogen.

The above notwithstanding, most people would agree that a certain level of drinking is socially acceptable. Although not always limited to social settings, this degree of drinking is nevertheless often referred to as *social* drinking. Images of social drinking abound in the media. The local sports bar gathering (or tailgate party), and the Friday afternoon happy hour are but a few examples.

At the other extreme of the drinking spectrum is what the *DSM-5* now calls a severe alcohol use disorder. The symptoms that define this disorder overlap a great deal with what was once called alcohol dependence. It is also what people have traditionally called alcoholism. Individuals with this disorder generally maintain a more or less constant level of alcohol in their bloodstreams and experience negative symptoms (such as agitation, anxiety, or sweating), along with strong cravings to drink, whenever that level approaches zero. Bill Wilson, who formed AA, is part of this group, and it is for these individuals that AA has by tradition existed. It is quite reasonable to assert that for these men and women, abstinence remains the only sane goal to pursue. Our research review here supports that. For these people the following are appropriate recovery goals:

- setting abstinence, as opposed to controlled drinking, as a goal
- getting active in AA by selecting a home group, getting a sponsor, and attending several meetings per week
- identifying oneself as a "recovering alcoholic" and a "member" of AA

That leaves us with a rather large middle zone between low-risk drinking and alcoholism. The *DSM-5* divides this zone into two subzones: mild and moderate alcohol use disorders. These two subzones need not be thought of as separated by sharp lines, but rather as blending into one another. This extended zone can accommodate a wide range of drinking behavior, from the individual who has "one toe," so to speak, in the mild alcohol use disorder zone, to another who is in the moderate zone "with both feet" yet is still not an alcoholic.

Another way to think of the drinking spectrum is that it illustrates how alcoholism is a chronic, progressive, and *insidious* disease. An individual does not simply step from one zone into another (anywhere on the drinking spectrum), but instead is much more likely to gradually slip further along the spectrum. It also accounts for why most men and women do not "connect the dots" and realize either that they have indeed shifted right on the spectrum, or see how their drinking has gradually affected them. Virtually all substance abuse professionals can attest that alcoholism typically follows a course through all the drinking zones.

Of course, there are those individuals who for one reason or another know that they are somewhere in the middle of the drinking spectrum; they may even acknowledge that they drink a lot yet choose to stay put. This group undoubtedly includes some of the heavy drinkers that Bill Wilson wrote about. There is not much we can say to such individuals other than to acknowledge that they are choosing of their own free will to live dangerously. I say this not based on personal opinion, but on an emerging body of hard evidence like the following.

A team of researchers from the University of Texas–Austin, the Palo Alto California Veterans Administration Hospital, and Stanford University set out to take a look at the health effects, including mortality, of heavy drinking versus moderate drinking. They began by identifying men and women whose self-reported drinking placed them into one of two categories:

- *Regular moderate drinkers:* These were men and women whose drinking pretty much coincided with the NIAAA guidelines cited earlier: a maximum of seven drinks per week for women and fourteen drinks per week for men. In addition, these individuals stated that the maximum number of drinks they'd consumed on any one occasion in the prior month was less than four for women and less than five for men.

- *Heavy episodic drinkers:* These were men and women whose typical drinking behavior also conformed to NIAAA recommendations, but who also stated that the maximum number of drinks they'd consumed on any one occasion in the prior month was more than four for women and more than five for men.

To sum up, the second group were men and women who were not regular heavy drinkers, in the sense of daily use, but who did drink fairly heavily on occasion—specifically, at least once a month.

In addition to assessing their drinking, the researchers also evaluated the entire group at the outset for these factors: medical conditions, obesity, smoking status, physical activity, and depression. They wanted to know, of course, if any of these other factors might affect the future health status and mortality of the two groups of drinkers.

This is another example of a longitudinal study, as the male and female subjects were followed for twenty years. Such studies stand to tell us a lot about the effects of anything—in this case drinking—because they shed light on long-term as opposed to short-term outcomes.

In this case, the results should give pause to everyone who considers themselves not a moderate drinker, but an episodic heavy drinker. Keep in mind that this latter group does not fall at the extreme right on the drinking spectrum—they are not alcoholics. The various up-front assessments revealed lower rates of obesity, smoking, and depression for the regular moderate drinkers than the men and women who were episodic heavy drinkers. These are called *covariates*, and their inclusion might make one lean toward an interpretation that smoking, obesity, or depression might account for any long-term health consequences among the episodic heavy drinkers. But that was not what the data analysis revealed. Here are the results in the researchers' own words:

> After adjusting for all covariates, as well as overall alcohol consumption, moderate drinkers who were episodic heavy drinkers showed a more than 2 times increase in the odds of total mortality during the 20-year period. Findings did not differ for women and men.

Now that should get our attention: episodic heavy drinking trumps obesity and smoking when it comes to mortality! It also brings to mind a piece of data we went over earlier, that the NIAAA guidelines for "low-risk drinking" need to be seen in context. The man who has two beers a night for seven nights is consuming fourteen beers per week, which falls within the NIAAA guidelines for a low-risk regular drinker. But what about the man who consumes seven beers two nights a week? He fits the criteria for an episodic heavy drinker. As such, this research informs us, he is twice as likely to die in a twenty-year period as a result of his drinking *pattern,* not the total amount that he consumes.

There are many people today who regularly drink in excess of the low-risk level but who rarely if ever binge or get really drunk. Depending, though, on just how far into even the mild alcohol use disorder zone they may be (one toe, a foot, two feet?), they may eventually begin to experience some subtle consequences related to drinking. They may experience disrupted sleep patterns, for example, leading in time to a loss of stamina. They may become less engaged in their closest relationships. Or they may be told that their performance at work is not up to par. If they should slip further—toward the moderate alcohol use disorder zone— others close to them are likely to connect the dots between drinking and its consequences, but they themselves may still fail to make the connection. Consequently, they are also unlikely to be motivated to alter their drinking habits, unless and until a more serious drinking-related consequence befalls them. When asked by a loved one of such an individual (who has indeed connected the dots) for my best advice, I've suggested avoiding diagnostic terms of any kind (most of all the dreaded term *alcoholic*) and instead simply but repeatedly pointing out the connection.

Saying things like, "Have you noticed that since you started drinking more wine at night you tend to fall asleep a lot earlier than you used to?" could over time help to facilitate the kind of introspection that is often a prelude to change.

So, what about these individuals who gradually move just a little deeper into the alcohol use disorder zones? What, if anything, does our review of research yield to inform them? One way or another, some of these men and women will come to realize that drinking is causing some problems in their lives. But even if that happens, what should they do about it? The research we reviewed on Moderation Management indicated that MM appeals primarily to younger individuals (24 percent were under age thirty-five) whose drinking behavior falls considerably below that which is defined as *dependence* (*DSM-IV*) or *severe* (*DSM-5*). About half of these individuals are women and about 80 percent were actively employed; the majority were college educated, and they had a supportive social network. For this group, strategies aimed at moderation appear to be effective. This subgroup of drinkers was able to shift left on "the drinking world" spectrum above into a safer place.

With respect to behavioral self-control, another controlled drinking approach, the outcome of objective research was similar. If you recall, roughly 25 percent of those who started out in BSC eventually settled on abstinence as their goal, while 15 percent were successfully able to moderate their drinking.

While it seems clear that strategies aimed at moderation may indeed work for some people who have experienced drinking-related problems, a careful and honest self-evaluation is probably the best starting point. Remember, researchers noted that about 15 percent of MM members reported experiences that suggest they were actually much deeper into the problem drinking zone.

These experiences included blackouts when drinking, tremors when not drinking, intense cravings to drink, and even convulsions. It could be said that men and women in this group are in "denial" about the extent of their drinking problem, and it would be misguided for professionals to advocate moderation strategies as a solution.

Looking again at the spectrum that represents the drinking world, we might ask: What about people whose drinking pattern places them somewhere to the right of the light gray "mild problem drinking" zone but still short of the black "severe problem drinking" zone? In particular, what if anything should a responsible professional advise these people to do concerning their drinking or drug use? Should professionals advocate for abstinence as the best goal for this group and, therefore, seek to facilitate their active involvement in a Twelve Step fellowship?

To answer these questions, it is once again probably wise for people in this wide zone of drinking or drug use to begin with a personal inventory (perhaps with the help of a counselor) of the consequences that have accrued in their lives that can be traced to drinking or drug use. In such a review it is important to keep in mind that because they have most likely moved into this zone gradually over a period that can easily span years, these individuals may very well be oblivious to the extent of their substance use and its consequences. That's not to say they are in denial; rather, they may simply be unaware of how substance use has progressively affected them.

Here are some areas that should be given a fresh look during a personal inventory:

- *Physical health:* Physical health typically deteriorates slowly as drinking moves from low-risk through the mild zone and into the moderate zone. Moreover, some physical ailments may be falsely attributed to the aging process, especially if health care professionals do not inquire about their patients' drinking habits. Research supports this: while most primary care providers ask patients about their drinking, only 13 percent use any kind of screening tool, even though many of these are brief and readily available.

In addition to contributing to diseases such as diabetes, pancreatitis, and hypertension, alcohol consumption has been directly linked with many forms of cancer as well as heart attacks. Women appear to be more vulnerable than men to many of these diseases simply because of the way their bodies metabolize alcohol.

Finally, accidents and falls are common at this zone of the drinking spectrum, as are visits to an emergency room or a walk-in clinic for such injuries.

- *Mental health:* According to the National Institute on Alcohol Abuse and Alcoholism, many patients are misdiagnosed with depression and treated with antidepressants when the true cause of their depression is drinking. Alcohol is a central nervous system depressant, and when used regularly in quantities like those associated with the moderate drinking zone, it will often disrupt the sleep cycle, causing insomnia or disrupted sleep, with resulting loss of energy and stamina. These symptoms easily mimic depression. In time, cognitive deficits such as impaired memory can also develop from heavy drinking. And for some, alcohol increases the potential for violence and subsequent arrests.

- *Relationships:* As drinking gradually progresses further into the moderate zone, fatigue and lack of energy tend to interfere with normal social relationships. Less time, for example, may be spent with friends who either do not drink or drink little, in favor of friends who are also heavy drinkers. Involvement in family life may also wane, along with the fulfillment of household responsibilities. Arguing over drinking becomes more common when drinkers are in this zone.

- *Work or school performance:* Declining work or school performance may be slow to be recognized as related to drinking, especially if that drinking is limited to after-hours. In addition, students may shield declining grades from parents, just as adults may work to keep their significant others from learning about poor performance ratings on the job. That said, individuals will surely know if their performance at school or at work has declined—even though they may attempt to blame others, as opposed to drinking, for these outcomes.

- *Financial:* Financial consequences related to increased drinking may include more money spent on liquor (or in bars), but they may also include lost or declining wages, such as bonuses or raises, that are actually the result of poor performance on the job. Beyond that, many men and women incur substantial legal costs associated with arrests for DUI.

The above are some of the more common consequences associated with movement further right on the "the drinking world" spectrum. Generally speaking, these men and women have not yet experienced the most severe physical symptoms of alcohol dependence. Some may have had one or more blackouts, frequent hangovers, and so on. They may have experimented with one or more "morning after" remedies. They may have had their share of bumps and bruises, or stitches. Yet surprisingly, many are able to maintain some degree of work performance and family life, even if these are not what they once were. These individuals—like Caroline Knapp—are sometimes referred to as "high-functioning alcoholics," which may be an apt term in many cases.

Unlike those who land further to the left on the drinking spectrum, these individuals would be well advised to pursue either total abstinence or conditional abstinence for a minimum of ninety days, as their goal. In the research we've looked at, conditional abstinence as a personal goal has been found to be generally inferior to complete abstinence, and that is certainly the case for people diagnosed as alcohol dependent using the traditional diagnostic criteria. For those who fall short of this, some re-evaluation following a significant period of abstinence may be reasonable. Of course, much would depend on what happens then. For example, if an individual is unable to abstain for ninety days despite several attempts, or abstains for ninety days but then promptly resumes drinking and in short order returns to the same old habits, then abstinence looms more and more as the most appropriate goal.

Summing Up

In this chapter, we examined the great abstinence debate that has largely driven criticism of AA and its Twelve Step program of recovery for many years. The concept of controlled drinking may indeed have its place, though research tells us that it is for a select group of individuals whose drinking problems fall on the milder side of the "drinking world," as we have defined it based on a new diagnostic schema developed by the American Psychiatric Association. We have seen how the drinking goal set by an individual—abstinence or controlled drinking—can exert a strong influence on outcome. We have also learned that one's personal identity—particularly as a recovering alcoholic and a member of AA—also has powerful effects. Finally, for those who choose to pursue abstinence, active efforts by a therapist to facilitate involvement in a Twelve Step fellowship leads to superior outcomes.

Food for Thought

1. Have you used any of the following of William R. Miller's behavioral self-control measures to help maintain abstinence?

   • goal-setting

   • self-monitoring

   • self-reinforcement

   • identifying high-risk situations

   • finding alternatives to drinking to deal with stress

   If not, do you think they might help?

2. How would you rate yourself on the following motivation for recovery statements, using a scale of 1 to 6? (1 is "strongly disagree"; 6 is "strongly agree")

   • Staying sober is the most important thing in my life.

   • I am totally committed to staying off alcohol/drugs.

3. Assessing the impact of your drinking on your physical health, mental health, relationships, work or school performance, and finances, where would you place yourself on "the drinking world" spectrum?

The Drinking World

Alcoholic

Low Risk "Social" Drinking	Mild Problem Drinking	Moderate Problem Drinking	Severe Problem Drinking

© Harvard University 2012

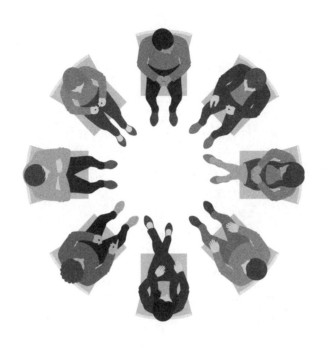

PART 2
How It Works

The Dynamics of Recovery I
Social Networks and Recovery

The research we reviewed in part 1 on AA and recovery can lead to only one reasonable conclusion: "if you work it, it works." *Working it* means getting involved in meetings, finding a sponsor, identifying oneself with AA, working its Twelve Step program, reading materials relevant to recovery, and so on. In effect, working it means being on the inside, looking out, as opposed to being on the outside, looking in—which may describe many of the people who claim that the Twelve Step program hasn't worked. Even before many of the studies discussed in part 1 were implemented, a group of researchers from numerous major research centers decided in 2004 to write a consensus article stating their shared opinion on the efficacy of self-help groups. The most ubiquitous of these of course is AA, but also included were fellowships that, like AA, share abstinence from alcohol and drugs as their goal. These fellowships include the following:

Al-Anon Family Groups (which offers support for significant others of substance abusers)

Narcotics Anonymous

Cocaine Anonymous

Marijuana Anonymous

Oxford House

Nicotine Anonymous

Secular Organizations for Sobriety

Double Trouble in Recovery

SMART Recovery

Women for Sobriety

Dual Recovery Anonymous

Dual Diagnosis Anonymous

The above vary a great deal with respect to their availability, but they all advocate abstinence as a goal and offer support and advice to their members for maintaining it. After reviewing the available research, this prominent group collectively reached the following conclusion, which was published along with its review in the *Journal of Substance Abuse Treatment*:

> Addiction self-help organizations are a major resource for addicted individuals, as well as for those who treat addicted people, work with them, and care about them. Research to date suggests that self-help groups can be beneficial, but also cautions that we have much more to learn about how they work and how they can be supported through clinical, agency, and policy actions.

Much research has taken place since the above policy statement was issued, and it supports the contention that these organizations are helpful, not only to people with substance use disorders, but also to those who work with them and those who love and care about them. The authors correctly point out that more needed to be done in understanding just how these fellowships help, and that is the subject here in part 2. They also suggest that more work was needed to determine how clinicians can effectively promote the use of self-help groups and Twelve Step fellowships. Some of this work has since been done and was reported in chapter 3, where two therapies in particular—MAAEZ and TSF—were discussed. That research found that therapists' efforts directed specifically at facilitating Twelve Step fellowship involvement were connected to superior outcomes with respect to two standard measures: days abstinent and drinks per drinking day. Other studies showed that setting a goal of abstinence, as opposed to either controlled drinking or "temporary" abstinence, was also associated with better outcome on these measures, as well as on "days to relapse."

In this chapter and the ones that follow, we will explore research related to another key issue raised in the above policy statement: exactly *how* Twelve Step fellowships help. To explore that question, we will focus on one aspect of Twelve Step recovery at a time. In this chapter we look at social support and the role it plays in recovery.

Social Support and Recovery

Project MATCH, discussed earlier in our review of therapies for alcohol use disorders, was a highly ambitious and carefully designed study that yielded an immense amount of data that have been analyzed by numerous researchers working at different academic institutions. To the extent that these researchers' findings converge, or agree, it strengthens their conclusions.

Let's begin with two studies from two different research centers, both of which sought to shed light on this question: do individuals whose social networks tend to support or encourage drinking do better or worse in different kinds of treatment?

Project MATCH, you may recall, utilized three different treatments, one of which (Twelve Step Facilitation or TSF) was aimed specifically at facilitating involvement in AA. One of the other treatments (cognitive behavioral therapy or CBT) sought to teach individuals skills they could use to resist urges to drink, cope with stress, and so on; the third (motivational enhancement therapy, or MET) aimed to enhance individuals' motivation to do something about their drinking.

Two different research teams, at two different times, explored this issue: for men and women with alcohol use disorders, how do the people they associate with influence their recovery? One study looked at how social networks affect men and women one year after completing treatment; the other looked at the effects three years post-treatment. We'll look at these in reverse order, since the three-year follow-up study was conducted nine years before new researchers took a fresh look at the data.

Richard Longabaugh is a professor of psychiatry and human behavior at Brown University Medical School. He is a fellow of the American Psychological Association, and in 1999 he was the recipient of the Dan Anderson Research Award from the Hazelden Foundation. For many years, he led the Center for Alcohol and Addiction Studies at Brown.

Longabaugh collaborated with colleagues at George Washington University, the University Wisconsin–Milwaukee, and Butler Hospital in Providence, Rhode Island, to discern how 806 individuals diagnosed as alcohol dependent were doing three years after being randomly assigned to and completing one of the three treatments tested in Project MATCH. Remember, of these treatments, two do not advocate for AA or even recommend it, while TSF purposefully facilitates and promotes active involvement in AA through a combination of education, discussion, and coaching.

Defining AA Involvement

"Involvement," if you recall from our earlier discussion of TSF treatment, means more than just being there, just attending AA meetings, even though a person's recovery may begin with that simple act of walking through the door of an AA meeting.

If we were to accept attendance alone as a measure of involvement, then we could just ask participants in studies like MATCH how many meetings they've attended, say in the past thirty days, and then correlate that with measures such as how many days they were abstinent during that time and how much they drank if they did drink. But that would only scratch the surface when it comes to involvement, as attested to, for example, by AA's own triennial membership surveys. To measure involvement more accurately, researchers at the University of New Mexico developed a measure they named the Alcoholics Anonymous Involvement Scale (AAI). Its principal developer is J. Scott Tonigan, PhD, a research professor in the university's Department of Psychology and its Center on Alcoholism, Substance Abuse, and Addictions (CASAA). He has a strong interest in understanding the dynamic forces within the AA fellowship that help to make it work.

The AAI is a thirteen-item inventory that asks questions like the following:

Have you attended an AA meeting in the last year?

Have you ever considered yourself to be a member of AA?

Have you ever gone to ninety AA meetings in ninety days?

Have you ever celebrated a sobriety birthday?

Have you ever had an AA sponsor?

Have you ever been an AA sponsor?

Have you ever had a spiritual awakening or conversion experience since your involvement in AA?

The items in the AAI represent a way to measure AA involvement on a graduated scale that ranges from minimal involvement to fairly intense involvement.

Defining Network Support

Broadly speaking, "network support for drinking" refers to how much and how often a person's close circle of family and friends consume alcohol. To measure it, individuals are asked to identify those friends, co-workers, or family members who they feel are most important in their lives. The individual then rates each person with respect to how often and how much he or she drinks. Finally, the individuals in the support network are rated with respect to how much they support (are in favor of) drinking. In this way, people who enter treatment have specific knowledge about whether those closest to them will likely support their recovery (abstinence from drinking) or support continued drinking.

The first finding of significance from this ambitious and sophisticated study was that, three years following treatment, those individuals assigned to TSF, whose goal is to facilitate active involvement in AA, reported being abstinent more than 80 percent of the time even when their social support network favored drinking. In other words, if a person's closest associates tend to drink and have a tolerant or even encouraging attitude toward drinking, then treatment that encourages involvement in a fellowship that supports sobriety can help counterbalance the influence of that social network.

In comparison, the percent of days abstinent for the other two treatments (CBT and MET) ranged from 65 to 70 percent. On the one hand—and this is good news—these data are encouraging in that they indicate that all three treatments were fairly effective. After all, being sober 65 percent of the time as long as three years after treatment could hardly be considered a failure. On the other hand, the data also point strongly to the influence that social support networks exert. AA is a social support network—one that supports sobriety, not drinking—and this study found that associating with AA led to significantly better outcomes. In addition, as noted earlier, many of those who received CBT or MET stated that they also voluntarily attended AA meetings.

There is another significant finding from this study that warrants a closer look. That has to do with what is called the *interaction* between AA involvement and network support for drinking. Another question the researchers were looking to answer is this: does the degree of involvement in AA matter? That is, how much difference does milder versus stronger involvement in AA make with respect to outcome? If a person's social network is made up primarily of drinkers, does it help to be deeply involved in AA?

Because they collected data that allowed them to assess just how supportive of drinking (versus sobriety) a person's social network was, as well as how involved that person was in AA, the researchers could use statistical analyses to shed light on this question. What they found was that greater involvement in AA had an *inoculation* effect. Put simply, the more involved people were in AA, the better their outcome at the three-year mark when their social network was most supportive of drinking. Those people who were most involved in AA, as defined above, were sober more than 90 percent of the time, even when their closest family and friends tended to be drinkers. In comparison, those who were less engaged in AA were sober a little less than 60 percent of the time when their social networks were similarly supportive of drinking.

This study is very significant because it strongly suggests that AA and its Twelve Step program works, in part, because greater involvement in AA contributes to a more resilient recovery, in the sense of being more resistant to outside social influences.

The concept of replication and why it is important in research was discussed earlier, and it is again relevant here. Much of the evidence presented in this book is based on data that have been found to be true not just once, or by a single researcher, but rather by researchers working in collaboration on studies that have been replicated. It represents not a one-off result, but a convergence of a large body of research findings.

The study we'll look at now falls into this category of replication, but with a bit of a twist. It was conducted by psychologists at the University of Illinois–Chicago. They followed 952 individuals who had been randomly assigned to one of the three different treatments of this project. Again, the question was the same: would individuals whose personal social networks (family, co-workers, and friends) tended to be drinkers do better if they were assigned to a treatment program whose specific goal was to facilitate their involvement in the AA fellowship?

Rather than looking at abstinence, these researchers focused on *negative consequences associated with drinking*. For this they used an instrument with an interesting name: the Drinker Inventory of Consequences—Recent (DrInC). The DrInC, a fifty-item questionnaire, asks about consequences of drinking not in an individual's distant past, but in the relatively recent past. As such, this tool is useful in assessing the effectiveness of treatment for an alcohol use disorder.

Consequences assessed by the DrInC include the following:

- impulse control (such as driving under the influence)
- physical consequences (such as hangovers)
- intrapersonal reactions (such as feeling guilty)
- interpersonal consequences (such as relationship problems)
- social responsibility (such as absenteeism)

Using the DrInC, the researchers classified the 952 participants into three classes: low consequences, medium consequences, and high consequences. They were then able to look at consequences ranging from low to high and compare these to level of network support for drinking, also from low to high.

The results were striking. For those men and women whose treatment sought to enhance their involvement in AA, negative consequences associated with drinking were essentially zero, regardless of whether their personal social network ranked low, medium, or high on support for drinking. In contrast, for those who received treatments that did not seek to enhance AA involvement (or even recommend AA attendance, for that matter), drinking consequences were directly related to social support— the more their personal social network supported drinking, the more they reported negative consequences from drinking.

This study mirrors and reinforces the conclusion stated above: one of the dynamic factors that accounts for why AA and its Twelve Step program works is because greater involvement in that fellowship contributes to a more resilient recovery. In this case that resilience was measured in terms of how many negative drinking consequences an individual experienced.

The Network Support Project

A team of researchers led by Mark Litt, professor of behavioral sciences and community health at the University of Connecticut Health Center, was also interested in this issue of network support and its relation to recovery. They pursued and won funding for a study comparing three different approaches to treating men and women who had been diagnosed as alcohol dependent—or to use the new terminology, men and women with *severe alcohol use disorders*. They call their intervention the Network Support Project.

Litt and his colleagues devised three treatment regimens, each of which was conducted in twelve weekly, sixty-minute, one-to-one sessions. Here are brief descriptions of these treatments:

- *Case management (CM):* This is often also referred to as *treatment as usual.* It consists of the patient and therapist using a checklist to identify areas and issues that could be barriers to abstinence from drinking. These include family problems and conflicts, financial issues, medical problems, and emotional problems such as depression. The therapist and patient then work together to identify resources that can be brought to bear (referral to a psychiatrist for depression, for example) as well as other potential solutions to these barriers to abstinence.

- *Network support (NS):* This intervention was based largely on the Twelve Step Facilitation (TSF) intervention that has already been discussed. However, in addition to trying to facilitate involvement in AA as a social network supportive of sobriety, the therapist also actively promoted involvement in *any* social network that supported sobriety, such as family and friends who were not drinkers.

- *Network support plus contingency management (NS/CM):* In this treatment, therapists also employed modified TSF as described above. But in addition patients could earn rewards, ranging from a couple of dollars to twenty dollars or more, for showing that they had taken action between therapy sessions to develop a non-drinking social network. Patients who demonstrated that they had done some positive work in this area (for example, going to an AA meeting) would pick a slip of paper at random from a fishbowl. About half the slips indicated rewards; the others simply said, "Sorry, try again next time." Those who had engaged in more than one activity since the previous session to build their social network could earn additional drawings for rewards.

In their first published report, this group described results from the Network Support Project immediately following treatment. Let's look at these first results, beginning with the big picture, and then take a closer look at the details, which turn out to be interesting.

Of the three treatments, network support produced a consistently superior outcome. That is, those men and women who underwent the treatment designed to promote attendance at AA as well as increase the number of non-drinking friends in the individual's personal social network fared the best, as measured by both abstinence and negative consequences associated with drinking. This finding is yet more evidence in support of AA and its Twelve Step program, and even more specifically of the efficacy of building a social network that is supportive of abstinence. That, then, is the big picture; now for the interesting details.

The NS treatment was designed to encourage two things: attendance at AA and connecting socially with *non-drinking* friends, family members, and others. What the data showed was that these men and women by and large did not avoid their associates who drank; rather, they added a friend or two who did not drink to their social circle.

Adding even a single non-drinking friend to their social network helped, but not nearly as much as attending AA meetings. This led the researchers to conclude, "In many instances, AA was indeed being used as an additional social network." The message to therapists and counselors here is clear: It's good to encourage people who have significant alcohol use disorders, and for whom abstinence is the goal, to expand their social network to include non-drinkers; however, that in itself is not enough. If abstinence is the goal, it's not enough to add one or more new contacts who are supportive of abstinence to one's existing social network. A supportive fellowship is also needed. Though a number of abstinence-based fellowships exist and would appear to be appropriate for this purpose, AA is by far the most ubiquitous.

Another interesting conclusion that the researchers offer concerns the comparison between the two treatments that sought to enhance AA attendance (NS and NS/CM) and the one that didn't, case management. The researchers asked the patients in all three treatments about their AA attendance. In the NS and NS/CM conditions this was, of course, encouraged, but in the CM condition it was not. They found that 61 percent of those who received either the NS or its similar NS/CM treatment attended AA meetings regularly; further, for this group greater AA involvement led to better outcome. In contrast, only 18 percent of those who received the case management (CM) treatment attended AA and, as stated for this group, the outcome was not as good.

The researchers then concluded with the statement "Participants can be encouraged to self-select." In other words, AA involvement and the building of a supportive social network are both goals that can be facilitated through a therapy that specifically encourages those activities, in the belief that building a strong social network in favor of abstinence is a powerful dynamic underlying recovery.

This last conclusion may be relevant to a discussion that occurred earlier in this book about how many people drop out of AA after trying it for only a short time. Some have suggested that this means AA is ineffective. However, like the case management treatment used in this study (as well as the cognitive behavioral and motivational enhancement therapies used in other studies), AA does not have a "program" specifically designed to facilitate further involvement. Indeed, AA is neither a therapy nor a treatment. AA remains a *fellowship* that is based on attraction, with the level and manner of Twelve Step program adoption being entirely up to individual members, and it deliberately avoids creating any form of intervention that promotes AA involvement. The closest it comes to this might be its tradition of "welcoming the newcomer" and its statement that "the most important person at a meeting is the newcomer." But that does not mean that counselors and clinics who treat men and women with substance use disorders should take the same approach. On the contrary, armed with firm knowledge that "If you work it, it works," along with strategies aimed at facilitating

AA involvement, research overwhelmingly points to that active facilitation as an evidence-based treatment of choice.

Network Support Project: Two-Year Follow-Up
As in the previously discussed studies on network support, the research group at the University of Connecticut was interested not only in behavior immediately following treatment, but also in how patients were doing later on. Accordingly, they followed their group of 210 men and women (42 percent women) and re-assessed their drinking behavior twenty-seven months after treatment had ended. Here are highlights of what they found:

> Patients who received Network Support (NS) treatment reported an average of 80% abstinent days 2 years after treatment had ended, and 40% were reporting complete abstinence in the 90 days preceding their 2-year follow-up.

As was reported in the first publication on the Network Support Project, although the goal of network support treatment is to build a social network (made up of AA plus one's personal social circle) that supports sobriety, what actually happened was that the participants did not *decrease* the number of drinkers in their personal social circle but tended to *add* one or more non-drinkers to it. In this context, adding AA as an extended support network appears to be what made the most difference in outcomes.

It's worth noting that although the therapists who administered the case management treatment were not advocating AA or intentionally trying to enhance AA involvement, AA involvement increased over time for all three treatment groups. In other words, some men and women migrated into AA on their own (think of the statistics reported in AA's triennial surveys in chapter 1). The difference in this research was that *when AA involvement was a specific treatment goal*, that involvement increased significantly more. So once again AA by itself attracted participation, but that participation could be enhanced through a therapeutic intervention.

The Problem with Contingency Management

This group of researchers from the University of Connecticut included a third intervention that it labeled network support plus contingency management. This therapy was also intended to promote building a personal network supportive of recovery, to include both family and friends and AA. However, remember that in addition to recommending and following up on AA attendance and involvement, participants in this treatment arm could earn small rewards for that attendance and involvement.

The idea behind contingency management comes from classical behavior therapy and reflects the notion that people's behavior is influenced by reward and punishment—in this case reward. So giving participants rewards for attending AA meetings, reading AA materials, and doing other activities that promoted recovery was seen as another strategy to enhance AA involvement. But that is not the way it turned out.

As the authors note, the results of the NS/CM treatment were disappointing. As they put it, "Participants in the NS/CM condition initially did as well as those in NS but at the end of 2 years were reporting the same outcomes as those in case management." What happened?

The answer to why the strategy seemed to fall flat appears to lie in the concept of *self-efficacy* and how it might interact with a system of rewards like the one used in the contingency management treatment.

Basically, self-efficacy is psychological jargon for self-confidence. These researchers measured self-efficacy using something called the Alcohol Abstinence Self-Efficacy Scale (AASE), which was developed by Carlo DiClemente, PhD, and associates at the University of Maryland. DiClemente is a professor of psychology at the University of Maryland–Baltimore County. A renowned researcher as well as a theorist, he was the recipient of a Lifetime Achievement Award for his work in the area of addictions from the Association for Behavioral and Cognitive Therapies. He is perhaps best known in the professional community for his work with James Prochaska on the development of a model for understanding how people change. Their Stages of Change model is widely used by therapists to assess how ready individuals are to change and how they move from a point where they do not believe they have a problem (for example, with drinking) through various stages, culminating in a decision to do something to change their behavior.

The AASE reflects one of DiClemente's other interests: how self-efficacy, or self-confidence, influences behavior. It asks respondents to answer, on a scale of 1 to 5 (with 5 being the most confident), how confident they are that they could abstain from drinking in twenty different situations. Here is a sample of these situations:

- when I am feeling angry inside
- when I am feeling depressed
- when I see others drinking at a party
- when I am on vacation and want to relax
- when I am physically tired

The higher the score on the twenty-item AASE, the more self-confident the individual is that his or her recovery is robust enough to resist drinking.

As noted above, in the Network Support Project, the contingency management (reward) treatment led to improvements in drinking initially, but these improvements had tapered off within two years. In contrast, the data on self-efficacy showed that at the two-year mark, the men and women who had received the contingency management treatment had *lower* self-efficacy scores than those who had received the network support treatment aimed at building a positive social support system (including AA), but without any external rewards like a raffle system for attending meetings.

Looking at these results, the researchers suggest that the reward system may actually have backfired. In order to maintain change—in this case, abstinence—individuals need to be able to attribute that change to themselves. In other words, the change needs to stem from their improved self-confidence as opposed to anything external, like a chance to win a $10 reward.

If the above answer to "what happened" makes sense, then clinics and clinicians would be wise to carefully consider whether or not to use any external incentives in treatment to motivate change. As an example, in some studies that this writer has been a consultant to, bus tokens and Walmart gift cards have been used to encourage both treatment attendance and AA participation. This would not appear to be the same as a raffle that offers random cash rewards or gift cards for attending AA meetings, yet it still needs to be monitored so that it does not appear to be a "pay for change" intervention. In studies where participants were actually paid for that participation, it's been my distinct impression that some were in it at least partly for the money and that any behavioral change was short-lived and prone to disappear promptly after the treatment ended.

The Influence of Heavy Drinkers in a Support Network

The last study we will review here involved 367 men and 288 women seeking treatment at ten public and private treatment programs in Northern California. The researchers in this case were interested in how both AA involvement and the participants' personal social networks might influence their recovery—specifically, abstinence. AA involvement again was measured not only in terms of the number of meetings attended, but also by reading AA material, having a sponsor and a home group, and so on.

Social networks were measured by asking participants how many heavy drinkers were in their social circle and how many people in their network were encouraging of less drinking or abstinence, including anyone they knew who was active in AA. This cohort of 655 men and women were followed for three years after treatment ended.

These researchers found, first, that AA involvement predicted sobriety, at one year and again at three years after treatment. Specifically, the rate of abstinence at the three-year follow-up for people who were active in AA was essentially the same as at the one-year follow-up. *Continued AA involvement supported ongoing recovery.* This finding challenges some in the treatment community who have expressed doubt about the value of ongoing AA involvement beyond one year following treatment.

A second finding of this study is also clinically significant, and it concerns the influence that an individual's social network exerts, independent of his or her involvement in AA. The researchers found that any increase in the number of *heavy* drinkers in that social network was associated with a decrease in the chances of staying sober. Conversely, a 10 percent increase in the number of people in a social network who are supportive of sobriety was associated with a comparable increase in the chances of staying sober. Finally, for every new problem drinker who was added to a social network between years one and three, two people supportive of sobriety would need to be added to "balance out" the effect.

Think about that. AA involvement clearly influences recovery—but so does one's personal social network. As the other research we've examined revealed, the influence of AA involvement is so strong, in fact, that it can effectively counterbalance a social network made up of friends or family who drink. But this study also tells us that AA involvement is not totally impervious to the influence of a social network, especially problem drinkers. *Problem drinkers in a person's social network exert a more powerful and negative influence on recovery than non-drinkers.*

The most important lesson from these studies on network support is this: while AA involvement may be the most powerful predictor of recovery, it is highly beneficial for therapists to work toward *minimizing* the number of heavy drinkers, while simultaneously *maximizing* the number of people supportive of recovery in a person's social network. For example, if clients are intensely resistant to using AA as a support network, therapists could alternatively emphasize the influence that support networks exert and then to attempt to facilitate social network change—from one that supports drinking to one that supports recovery. Even in that case, however, clinicians would be wise to keep in mind the findings from the Network Support Project, which found that while building a social network supportive of recovery had a positive effect on sobriety, it was not nearly as powerful as AA involvement.

Summing Up

The research we've examined in this chapter does not by any means represent the totality of research on how social networks affect recovery. However, the studies we've looked at represent what I consider to be the most carefully designed and rigorously implemented studies on this subject. Collectively, they make it abundantly clear that one answer to the question "How does it work?" lies in the influence that social networks exert. AA and other abstinence-based fellowships offer an alternative social support network to the one that typically surrounds the problem drinker—particularly those whose drinking behavior places them at or near the severe or extreme right side of the drinking spectrum.

Food for Thought

1. Identify the people in your social network, such as family members, friends, co-workers, club or religious affiliation members, members of your Twelve Step recovery groups (including your sponsor). How many of these people are drinkers? How many are problem drinkers?

2. What can you do to increase the number of people in your network who support abstinence?

3. On a scale of 1 to 5, with 5 being the highest, how would you rate your "self-efficacy"— confidence in your ability to take responsibility for your actions and follow-through on your commitments? What can you do each day to increase your sense of self-efficacy regarding your recovery program?

◆

The Dynamics of Recovery II
Spirituality and Sponsorship

The role of spirituality in AA and its Twelve Step program of recovery has long been the subject of controversy. It stems in large part from the inclusion of a God concept in many of the Twelve Steps, beginning with Step Three:

> *Made a decision to turn our will and our lives over to the care of God* as we understood Him.

References to God also appear in several other steps, such as Step Five:

> *Admitted to God, to ourselves, and to another human being the exact nature of our wrongs.*

And again in Step Six:

> *Were entirely ready to have God remove all these defects of character.*

And finally, in Step Eleven:

*Sought through prayer and meditation to improve our
conscious contact with God as we understood Him,
praying only for knowledge of His will for us and the
power to carry that out.*

Some people have chosen to reject AA based on what is commonly referred to as "the God thing" within Twelve Step fellowships. It has also led some people to characterize AA as a religion, though it is not. Religions are governed by dogma, which is delivered by designated clergy who are monitored, in turn, via an authoritative hierarchy. AA has none of these things.

Others have seen fit to identify AA with one or another specific religion, such as Christianity or Catholicism. But this misses the point of the deliberate insertion of the phrase *as we understood Him,* which significantly clarifies the nature of the "God" that the originators of AA incorporated into their vision of recovery from addiction. For those who are interested in history, that vision and its evolution are detailed in Ernest Kurtz's book *Not-God,* which is a history of AA.

Bill Wilson, the prime author of the Twelve Steps, remained an avowed agnostic throughout his life. It is no accident, for example, that chapter 4 of *Alcoholics Anonymous* bears the title "We Agnostics." Wilson clearly saw the root of his own alcoholism—and, he inferred, others'—in an inflated ego. He wrote, "Selfishness—self-centeredness! That, we think, is the root of our troubles," and "The alcoholic is an extreme example of self-will run riot." That insight was the inspiration for his epiphany: in order to overcome his alcoholism, Wilson needed to abandon egotism and self-will and instead reach out to others.

Viewed in the above context, it would appear that the AA Twelve Step program is one that urges humility above arrogance, along with a willingness to reach out to some "power" greater than individual willpower—a power greater than *self.* That power, which is referred to as God in the above Steps, is not, however, identified with any religion; rather, it is deliberately worded in a way that makes it a personal choice. Nevertheless, it speaks to the cornerstones of AA: reaching out as opposed to going it alone, collective support over individual willpower, humility over arrogance.

Spirituality has always been a core component of the AA program, but that spirituality is defined largely through its culture and traditions rather than by any specific religious dogma. This concept of spirituality is probably best expressed in the AA publication *Twelve Steps and Twelve Traditions.* We are left with the question, though, of whether spirituality itself, and therefore its role in recovery, can be studied using scientific methods. Happily the answer is that it can be, and has been studied in that way. We'll be looking at these studies shortly.

To put the concept of spirituality in context, it can also be helpful to view it in a larger cultural context. Surveys have found, for example, that 94 percent of Americans profess a belief in God or some other "Higher Power" that supersedes personal willpower. Almost half of these people attend religious services of some kind in any given week. And one in four state that they have turned to prayer for aid with an illness or other personal crisis at some point in the prior year.

These figures contrast sharply with surveys of psychiatrists and other mental health professionals. A majority of psychiatrists, for example, do not espouse a belief in God or a Higher Power. This may be one reason why carefully conducted and sound research on spirituality as it relates to both addiction and recovery are relatively rare. That aside, the resurgence of interest in AA that resulted from studies like Project MATCH has spurred some interest in looking at this issue of spirituality and how it might contribute to recovery.

Spirituality and Recovery

The first study we'll look at was conducted by Stephanie Carroll, PhD, of the California School of Professional Psychology. Carroll recruited a sample of 100 AA members (51 male) from twenty different AA groups in Northern California. Her goal was to evaluate the relationship between the spiritual practices of these individuals and their recovery. To do this, of course, she needed first to define *spirituality* in some way and then measure it.

Carroll defined spirituality in terms of Steps Eleven and Twelve of the AA program. Step Eleven recommends the practice of meditation and prayer, and Step Twelve has to do with altruism, or reaching out to other alcoholics. While these are not aspects of any specific religion, most would agree that these activities meet the criteria for being manifestations of what we commonly think of as spirituality.

The activities related to these Steps were measured using a questionnaire that Carroll devised. It asked respondents to indicate how often they engaged in each of a number of activities, from daily to yearly. Here are some of the activities that Carroll's questionnaire asked about:

- prayer
- meditation
- reading spiritual material (for example, daily meditations)
- spending time in nature (for example, hiking or camping)
- interacting with art (such as visiting a museum, painting, or drawing)

- attending a religious service
- greeting a newcomer at an AA meeting
- engaging in AA service activities
- engaging in non-AA community service activities
- volunteering to be a sponsor or temporary sponsor

In this sample of active AA members, more than half reported praying or meditating twice a day as well as reading some form of spiritual literature three times a week. Half also reported listening to music that they defined as spiritual, meaning that it was consistent with meditation or prayer, on a weekly basis. Half also said that they interacted with art in some way at least monthly. Interestingly, despite these spiritual activities, less than half of the sample reported attending formal religious services. On the other hand, 90 percent said they attended AA meetings at least twice a week. It would seem, then, that it was AA, rather than an organized religion, that was the driving force behind these spiritual activities.

Carroll's questionnaire also asked respondents to indicate their current length of sobriety, in years and months. She then compared that to how the men and women in the sample scored on her spirituality scale.

What Carroll found was that those activities most closely associated with Step Eleven—such as meditating, praying, reading spiritual literature, and communing with art or nature—were significantly correlated with length of sobriety. In other words, those who engaged in these spiritual activities had a more robust recovery. As in other studies, AA meeting attendance was also linked with better recovery, but the spiritual activities in and of themselves predicted longer recovery.

As for Step Twelve activities, the study did not find a strong correlation between them and length of recovery. This is somewhat surprising, as reaching out to others in an altruistic way, which is at the core of Step Twelve, would seem to qualify as a spiritual activity. In her conclusion, though, Carroll noted that these results should be interpreted cautiously, as "the definition of Step 12 work is open to interpretation and is difficult to measure." If we look closely at Step Twelve, we can see that this may indeed be the case:

> *Having had a spiritual awakening as the result of these steps, we tried to carry this message to alcoholics, and to practice these principles in all our affairs.*

While activities such as prayer, meditation, and even reading or listening to "spiritual" books or music appear to fall clearly into the category of spiritual activities, it's arguable whether or not being a sponsor does. Nevertheless, the results of at least this first study indicate that spirituality, as defined above, is an independent dynamic force that contributes to recovery.

In 1996 a team of researchers from Duke University used a measure of spirituality that was not designed for studying recovery from alcoholism, but which they felt was compatible with the AA concept of spirituality. This instrument—the Matthew Materialism and Spiritualism Scale, or MMSS—is divided into several subscales. This reflects its authors' belief that spirituality is not a monolithic entity; instead, it is a concept made up of different but related components. Accordingly, the MMSS yields scores that include the following areas:

- *God:* Assesses the belief in a God or some other Higher Power
- *Religion:* Assesses religious practices

- *Mysticism:* Measures the belief in mystical experiences such as epiphanies, spiritual awakenings, or visions
- *Spirits:* Measures the belief in the existence of spirits and an afterlife
- *Character:* Assesses one's belief in the value of altruism, unselfishness, and kindness

These researchers conducted two related studies using a sample of 62 active AA members (half were men; half were women) with an average of sixteen years of sobriety. Of these individuals, 47 percent reported attending AA meetings three times a week. They were compared to a group of 20 clergy (100 percent Christian) who were contacted primarily through the Duke University Divinity School. Finally, the test was given to a group of 61 people from the general population.

The results of this study are instructive. First, there were no significant differences in any of the score between the group that was in recovery and the group of clergy. Second, the people in the recovery group scored higher than the group of people from the population in general on two scales: mysticism and character. What might this mean?

For starters, these results strongly suggest that people who identify themselves with AA and report having been in recovery for some time espouse spiritual beliefs comparable to those of clergy. That in itself is evidence again that spirituality is a dynamic force in recovery and that AA is correct in its belief that spirituality is central to recovery.

But that is not all we have to learn from these data. The men and women in the recovering group strongly identified with the factors labeled mysticism and character. Their beliefs in these areas turned out to be comparable to those held by clergy. This tells us, first, that this group had a stronger belief than those in the general public in the possibility of having a life-changing experience, call it a spiritual awakening, a vision, or an epiphany. William R. Miller, who was mentioned earlier in connection with his development of motivational enhancement therapy, is also interested in this phenomenon, which he calls *quantum change.* His book of the same title is listed in the references.

These results also reveal that the recovering group had a stronger-than-average belief in the value of character, or the capacity to be altruistic, unselfish, and kind—in short, to be humble instead of arrogant and to care for the welfare of others.

Now we come to other interesting questions: Are the men and women who affiliate with AA and who follow its Twelve Step program more spiritual *to begin with,* or does their experience of "working the program" lead them to become more spiritual over time? Also, does a prior belief in mysticism (before becoming active in AA) increase the likelihood that a person in recovery will at some point experience the "spiritual awakening" spoken of in AA writings?

To answer questions like these definitively we would need to identify a group of people who have alcohol use disorders and who start out having comparable spiritual beliefs as measured by the MMSS. In one approach, half of that group would be assigned to a treatment aimed at facilitating their affiliation with AA and commitment to its Twelve Step program, while the other half would not. Then we would have to assess and compare the spiritual beliefs of the two groups, say, five years later. Such a study would on the surface seem to be impossible to implement. How could one responsibly recruit a group of men and women with substance use disorders and then deliberately direct them away from AA, given what the research here has taught us?

Another approach might be to simply take a large group of people with substance use disorders, assess them for spiritual beliefs, and then simply follow them for an extended period, identifying those who pursue recovery through AA versus those who do not. We could then compare the two groups relative to their spiritual beliefs and determine whether the group that pursues AA was more spiritual at the outset than the group that did not. Such a naturalistic longitudinal study has not yet been conducted.

Rather than taking either of the above two approaches, the Duke researchers opted to ask the recovering men and women in their initial study to take the MMSS again, only this time answering it as they believe they would have *before* their drinking problem developed. In other words, they were all asked to reflect, retrospectively, on what their beliefs were before they had a problem with alcohol and before they decided to turn to AA. Here is what the data showed:

- On the God, religion, and mysticism scales, women reported lower scores than males before they entered recovery but higher scores than males after they had been in recovery for a significant number of years.

- On the spirits scale, women's scores increased through recovery while men's scores stayed essentially the same.

- Both sexes indicate an increase on the character scale through recovery, but women's increases were greater.

- Despite the above differences for women versus men, both sexes reported significant increases in their scores on all of the MMSS scales over time in recovery.

This study does suffer from one weakness, which is that it relies on the subjects to accurately report their pre-recovery spiritual beliefs. Nevertheless, it does again point to the idea that spirituality and spiritual growth—especially in the areas related to personal values such as altruism and kindness, along with a belief in the reality and possibility of epiphanies—are a core part of the Twelve Step program. Moreover, these data strongly suggest that it is AA involvement that supports such spiritual growth, as opposed to the idea that spiritually inclined men and women are naturally drawn to AA. The study results are also consistent with the findings of the Carroll study we looked at earlier.

As we move on in this examination of research on the role of spirituality in AA and recovery, it is instructive to consider the following statement that appears in an appendix of the AA Big Book.

> The terms "spiritual experience" and "spiritual awakening" are used many times in this book which, upon careful reading, shows that the personality change sufficient to bring about recovery from alcoholism has manifested itself among us in many different forms. . . .
>
> Though it was not our intention to create such an impression, many alcoholics have nevertheless concluded that in order to recover they must acquire an immediate and overwhelming "God-consciousness" followed at once by a vast change in feeling and outlook.
>
> Among our rapidly growing membership . . . such transformations, though frequent, are by no means the rule.

Although epiphanies appear to be a true phenomenon, here the author describes how, for many, a "spiritual awakening" occurs not as a sudden epiphany but rather as a significant shift in one's outlook on life that takes place gradually over time. This may be an important qualification, since my own impression from interviewing people in long-term recovery is that sobriety—as opposed to heavy drinking—inevitably affects an individual in a number of ways. On a physical level, the person feels better—more energized and vital, less stagnant and lethargic. That in turn allows the person to view social, family, and work situations from this new perspective, and perhaps to set new goals to pursue now that some energy and clarity of mind have returned. On a psychological level, recovery sets the stage for the emotional relief that many report when they are able to acknowledge the negative effect that alcohol has had on their lives, and how much better it is to be sober. In addition, acknowledging the "harm done" as a result of drinking and attempting to "make amends" where appropriate offers relief from guilt and shame. Looking at these effects of recovery in their totality, it isn't hard to imagine how together they make for the "personality change" described above or how that might amount to a "spiritual awakening."

AA Involvement, Abstinence, and Spirituality

A team of researchers headed by John Kelly of the Department of Psychiatry at Massachusetts General Hospital and Harvard Medical School, also decided to venture into this relatively little-studied concept of spirituality and what role it might play in recovery. Using a large sample of 1,726 men and women who had undergone treatment for alcohol use disorders, they looked at three variables:

- *Alcohol use:* They used the standard measures of percent days abstinent (PDA) and drinks per drinking day (DDD). PDA, to review, indicates the extent to which an individual abstains totally from alcohol, while DDD measures how many drinks a person consumes on a day when having a "slip."

- *AA attendance:* This was a simple measure, not of AA *involvement,* as was described earlier, but simply how many AA meetings an individual attended in the previous ninety days.

- *Spirituality:* To gauge spirituality, these researchers employed a measure called the Religious Background and Behavior (RBB) questionnaire. The RBB is worth a closer look, to see exactly how its authors define spirituality.

The RBB was developed by Gerard Connors of the Research Institute on Addictions and J. Scott Tonigan and William R. Miller of the University of New Mexico. They used a combination of self-identification along with an inventory of specific activities and experiences to capture and quantify the extent to which spirituality plays a role in an individual's life. For example, people taking the RBB are first asked to identify themself as one of the following:

- *Atheist:* Does not believe in God
- *Agnostic:* Believes we can't really know about God
- *Unsure:* Doesn't know what to believe about God
- *Spiritual:* Believes in God but is not religious
- *Religious:* Believes in God and practices a religion

Next, individuals taking the RBB are asked to estimate how often they engage in different activities on an eight-point scale that ranges from "never" to "more than once a day." The activities listed include

- praying
- meditating
- attending religious services
- reading holy or spiritual writings

If you recall, in her study of spirituality and recovery, Stephanie Carroll found that recovering men and women showed significant increase in spiritual beliefs that was correlated with AA involvement, yet less than half of them attended formal religious services. In their study, Kelly and colleagues found that higher scores on the spirituality/religiousness scale were positively related to PDA (abstinence) and negatively related to DDD (drinking). In other words, people who reported stronger spiritual beliefs were indeed more likely to remain abstinent and to drink less if they did slip.

In addition to the above, these researchers found that *spirituality/religiousness increased as their subjects attended more AA meetings over time.* This, too, suggests that it is active involvement in AA that gradually has the effect of promoting spiritual beliefs. Here is what the authors conclude on this topic:

> Results from this study, using a large multi-site clinical sample, exhibiting a broad range of alcohol-related involvement and impairment, support the central idea espoused by AA that spirituality is important in recovery and that AA appears to mobilize spiritual changes, which help explain AA's beneficial effects on recovery from alcohol dependence.

Although many people hold the view that spirituality is too vague a concept to quantify and study scientifically, I believe that we can draw several conclusions from the research we've looked at so far. The first is that, because AA emphasizes spirituality, those who identify with AA and work its program by and large do become more "spiritual" over time. Second, that spiritual growth itself contributes in a positive way to sustained recovery. Third, spirituality, as it is reflected in AA's emphasis on honesty, humility, and personal renewal, as opposed to formal religious observance, may be the key dynamic responsible for this change.

AA's focus on "character" and the capacity for honest self-appraisal, followed by a willingness to admit to faults and flaws, is easily construed as a program of character growth. When I, at least, ask individuals in recovery to think about those men and women who have influenced them the most, their descriptions invariably boil down to this thing we call character.

Working the Steps and Spirituality

One last study we should look at in our discussion of the role of spirituality in recovery comes from a group at the Center on Alcoholism, Substance Abuse, and Addictions (CASAA) at the University of New Mexico. This group wanted to examine what it calls "the general alcoholics anonymous tools of recovery" and it identified these tools with what is commonly referred to as "working the Steps" in the AA culture.

To begin, these researchers developed a questionnaire—which they aptly named the General Alcoholics Anonymous Tools of Recovery, or GAATOR—to elicit responses from men and women in recovery about how they personally work the Steps.

The GAATOR consists of twenty-four items, each of which is worded to closely model one of the Twelve Steps. Here are a few examples:

- I have turned my will and life over to my Higher Power. (Step Three)
- I have prayed and meditated. (Step Eleven)
- I have made a list of my resentments. (Step Four)
- I have made direct amends to those whom I have harmed. (Step Nine)

Men and women taking the GAATOR are asked to respond to each of its twenty-four statements as follows:

- false or definitely false = 0
- true or definitely true = 1

Theoretically, then, the GAATOR can yield scores ranging from 0 to 24 (though few fall at either extreme). The CASAA researchers administered it to 130 men and women (46 percent female) who indicated that they had *only recently* started attending AA meetings. At that initial point, this group reported drinking on average 44 percent of the previous ninety days and drinking an average of fourteen drinks every day that they drank. Without a doubt, this was a group of men and women who drank heavily. They were also ethnically and demographically diverse. This group was not assigned to any formal treatment, though if individuals asked they would be given contact information for local treatment facilities.

The entire group took the GAATOR at the outset of their involvement with AA and again three, six, and nine months later. The researchers then employed a statistical technique called *factor analysis* to determine how the various "tools" for working the Steps related to each other and how they related to drinking behavior. What they found was that the twenty-four GAATOR items formed two "clusters." One of these clusters consisted of questions that related to what we've already talked about as the spiritual components of the Twelve Steps. These include statements reflecting Steps One, Two, Three, Six, Seven, and Eleven, meaning that they refer to concepts and behaviors such as a belief in a Higher Power that is stronger than personal willpower, and using prayer and meditation as spiritual tools.

The second cluster consisted of statements that reflected what the researchers labeled the "behavioral" aspects of the Twelve Steps. That is, they felt these Steps referred to some form of *behavior*—to doing something. Included in this second cluster are Steps Four, Five, Eight, Nine, Ten, and Twelve, which concern things like conducting a personal moral inventory and making amends (when appropriate) for harm done to others as a consequence of drinking.

Here the researchers discovered that higher rates of AA meeting attendance plus treatment were associated with more spiritual Step work. Remember that the participants in this study were not required to enter treatment; however, the group that chose to do so ended up attending more AA meetings and consequently reported doing more spiritual Step work. This is completely consistent with findings we already examined and reinforces the notion that getting more involved in AA activities facilitates character change, or what is commonly referred to as spiritual growth. Keep in mind, however, that such spiritual growth has more to do with ethics and values than it does with any formal religious practices.

And what of the behavioral dimension? Well, that brings us to yet another dynamic force within the AA program of recovery, and that is *sponsorship*.

Sponsorship and Recovery

The idea of sponsorship dates to the very beginnings of AA, when it was indeed a small group of men who had discovered that by reaching out to one another and thereby placing their faith in some power greater than their personal willpower (which had failed them time and again), they had more success staying sober. In the early days of AA, a sponsor could easily be a man who'd been sober for a very short period of time but who was willing to escort a fellow drunk from the hospital to a meeting.

Today sponsorship remains a core component of the Twelve Step culture, though it has evolved somewhat. Nowadays, a sponsor is generally expected to be someone of the same sex (or sexual orientation) as the "sponsee." The sponsor is also expected to have been in recovery for some time (generally at least a year), to attend meetings regularly, to have a home group, and to have a sponsor of his or her own. In keeping with AA tradition and culture, no one need formally apply to be a sponsor, nor does the person necessarily have to meet all of these expectations. In the end, the decision is left to the individual sponsee and sponsor.

Newcomers to AA are encouraged to ask, as soon as possible, for a "temporary sponsor" who will help them understand the rules of the road at AA meetings, identify appropriate meetings to attend, and explain key AA concepts. A temporary sponsor will also typically ask the newcomer to check in frequently, through phone calls, emails, or text messages. Many sponsors arrange to meet face-to-face with their sponsee on a regular basis.

These activities clearly help cement the sponsor-sponsee bond, which for many is a bedrock of recovery, and encourage deep *involvement* in AA at this critical early stage of recovery.

At some point later on, an established AA member may decide to change sponsors, usually choosing someone he or she knows well and already has a friendship with. This is common and perfectly acceptable within the AA culture. In this subsequent relationship, the sponsor often helps the sponsee to "work the Steps" of the AA program of recovery.

Sponsorship within Twelve Step fellowships is intended to work both ways. For the sponsee, it is a source of one-to-one support, comfort, and advice rooted in experience. By checking in regularly, newcomers get support for "sticking with the program" despite urges to use, anxieties about the AA program, doubts about their ability to stay clean and sober, and even slips. The sponsor is neither a therapist nor a spiritual adviser, but is simply someone who has "walked the same path," struggled for recovery, and achieved some success. A temporary sponsor will typically encourage a newcomer to make other AA contacts, thereby facilitating an expanded social network supportive of recovery. In time the sponsor will be one—but not necessarily the only—person a sponsee can call if he or she feels in crisis, in danger of drinking, or has had a slip.

Sponsorship also works for the sponsor, as it represents an act of altruism that is consistent with the spiritual part of AA's message and its Twelfth Step. In AA parlance, sponsorship amounts to "Giving back to get" and "To keep it [sobriety, serenity, and so on], you have to give it away."

What light, if any, can research shed on sponsorship itself and its role in recovery? To begin to answer this question, we return to the study we just looked at. Those researchers, you'll recall, developed and used an instrument called the GAATOR (General AA Tools of Recovery) that identifies and measures two kinds of "Step work"—spiritual and behavioral. Spiritual Step work is said to take place when an individual AA member works on those Steps, such as Step Eleven, that advocate for meditation and prayer as a part of recovery.

In contrast, behavioral Step work is associated with those Steps that involve doing something. Step Nine, for example, which involves making amends, would fall into the behavioral category of Step work. Statistical analyses show that spiritual Step work and behavioral Step work tend to be independent—one can engage in one more than the other (or both equally).

The participants in this study were asked, as in many of the studies we've reviewed here, to provide information on how active they were in AA as relative newcomers to the program, including whether or not they had a sponsor. The researchers found that those who reported having a sponsor also tended to have higher scores on behavioral Step work. Having a temporary sponsor, however, was not associated with increased spiritual Step work.

It would appear, based on the above, that sponsorship is indeed an active ingredient, at least in early recovery, especially when it comes to doing things, like taking a moral inventory and making amends. Based on this initial study of these two dimensions of Step work, sponsorship has less influence when it comes to engaging in spiritual Step work such as prayer, meditation, or believing in a Higher Power. But remember that this applies to men and women in *early* recovery. The dynamics within a sponsor-sponsee relationship may change when recovery becomes more established and secure and the sponsee has worked more of the Steps. Nevertheless, AA has always identified itself as a program of action, and these findings suggest that sponsorship does indeed facilitate that action.

In a subsequent study, this same research group at CASAA decided to examine the issue of timing: how important it might be to have a sponsor *very early* on in recovery as opposed to *after* a person has been attending AA meetings for a while. In contrast to their previous study, which recruited men and women who had been active in AA but only for a relatively short period of time, now they would need to identify individuals who had just begun to attend AA and then follow them. Accordingly, for this study prospective participants were excluded if they met one of the following criteria:

- more than sixteen weeks of total lifetime exposure to AA
- abstinence from alcohol for twelve months or more after deciding that their drinking was a problem

Using these criteria, the researchers identify 253 eligible participants (62 percent male) who had alcohol use disorders but who were only beginning to utilize AA. They then used two measures we are by now familiar with:

- *Alcoholics Anonymous Involvement Scale (AAI):* The AAI is a measure not just of AA attendance but of AA *involvement,* including whether or not a person has a sponsor.
- *General Alcoholics Anonymous Tools of Recovery (GAATOR):* The GAATOR assesses the extent to which AA members are "working the Steps," including Steps that are identified as spiritual and Steps that are identified as behavioral (again, including sponsorship).

After being recruited into the study, these 253 men and women were followed for twelve months. They were asked to complete the above measures quarterly—at three months, six months, nine months, and twelve months. The results enabled the researchers to consider how behaviors such as having a sponsor might relate to recovery during this very early stage of abstinence. Moreover, they could then compare how having a sponsor very early on (months one to three) might compare to having waited to get a sponsor (for example, for four to six months) with respect to abstinence. Along the way, they could also look once more at whether AA involvement in general predicted recovery. This, of course, has been studied many times before—but as we know, replication is a good thing!

First, the results did in fact replicate (yet again) numerous other studies: that greater AA involvement—not just attendance—predicted increased abstinence. And increased abstinence, as reflected in the well-established criterion of percent days abstinent (PDA), is generally considered the gold standard in research. Its cousin, drinks per drinking day (DDD), is another frequently used outcome measure. In this study, increased AA involvement predicted higher PDA and lower DDD; in other words, more active AA members were more likely to remain abstinent and to drink less if they did have a slip.

Data like the above are consistent with the way AA has always described itself—as a fellowship whose sole criterion for membership is "a desire to stop drinking." In its writings, it also describes itself as a fellowship that "seeks progress rather than perfection." This is reflected in the AA culture itself, which celebrates recovery (one year, five years, and so on) but also accepts "slips" as well as full-blown "relapses" as part of the recovery process. AA culture emphasizes that members should do "the next best thing" following a slip, which is to contact an AA friend or sponsor and go to a meeting, where they will always be welcomed.

AA also recognizes addiction as a cunning disease that requires ongoing vigilance—through ongoing involvement in AA—as a means to contain it. Accordingly, outcome measures such as percent days abstinent and drinks per drinking day are totally appropriate when seeking to assess AA's effectiveness. As the studies reviewed here uniformly show, working the Twelve Steps—being active in AA—is associated with better outcomes.

But what about this issue of sponsorship? How important might timing be? This study sheds some interesting light on that. The researchers found that *having an AA sponsor early (within the first three months) increased the probability of complete abstinence at months four to six nearly threefold!* That is a pretty dramatic effect.

In contrast to the above, getting a sponsor later (in months seven to nine) did not predict abstinence at months ten to twelve. Does that mean that seeking out a sponsor later is useless? In my opinion, the answer to that is no. Although getting a sponsor early appears to reduce the risk of drinking, the adage "better late than never" may well apply here. Also, if you recall, the data we looked at in chapter 1, using AA's triennial member surveys, showed that about 80 percent of the respondents—regardless of how long they'd been clean and sober—indicated that they had a sponsor. It is entirely possible (perhaps likely) that the value of a sponsor-sponsee relationship changes over time. For example, it could be beneficial, once some recovery has been established, to have a sponsor when working the Steps on a deeper level. As an example, many men and women with substantial recovery will tell you that doing a "fearless moral inventory" six or eight months into recovery is a very different experience from doing it again six or eight *years* into recovery. The same goes for making amends.

One last study worth looking at for now recruited 495 men and women who sought treatment services for alcohol or other drug problems through a variety of treatment programs in a Northern California county. Nearly half were women and the average age of the group was thirty-eight. They were all evaluated before treatment and then again at one, three, five, and seven years following treatment. Longitudinal studies like this are important, as we've seen, because they tell us not just about how people do immediately after treatment, but what the trajectory of their recovery looks like years later as well as what factors might be related to better long-term outcomes.

This was a research team whose members were drawn from the Alcohol Research Group in Emeryville, California; the Karolinska Institute in Stockholm, Sweden; the School of Public Health at the University of California–Berkeley; and the University of California–San Francisco. Their study focused on two factors—AA attendance and the use of an AA sponsor—and examined how these factors might relate to abstinence. Theirs was a complex research design that divided abstinence, AA attendance, and sponsorship utilization each into a series of trajectories:

- *AA attendance:* Attendance at AA meetings was divided into these trajectories: *low* (five or six meetings a year on average), *medium* (an average of sixty meetings per year), and *high* (an average of five meetings per week in the first year, declining to an average of two per week by year seven).

- *Sponsorship:* Participants' responses were again divided into trajectories: *low* (only a 4 percent chance or less of having an AA sponsor at year seven) and *high* (a 75 percent chance of still having a sponsor at year seven).

- *Abstinence:* The abstinence trajectories included *low* (abstinence average 12 percent of the time across the seven years) and *high* (abstinence average of 75 percent in year one to almost 100 percent in year seven).

Here is what these researchers found, tracking participants' responses across years one through seven:

- Individuals classified as medium and high in terms of meeting attendance all had higher odds of remaining abstinent—four times as high for the high attendance group and over twice as high for the medium attendance group.

- Individuals in the high sponsorship group were seven times more likely to remain abstinent than those in the low sponsorship group.

- Study participants who maintained a sponsor over time had an added advantage over the group that no longer had a sponsor by year seven.

- Having an AA sponsor provided an advantage with respect to abstinence over and above meeting attendance alone.

- Greater AA meeting attendance in early recovery provided an advantage over those whose initial attendance rates were lower.

What lessons can be drawn from this final study? First, it points again to the advantage the would-be recovering person has if he or she gets a sponsor and keeps one (albeit not neces-sarily the same sponsor for seven years). Second, it confirms the advantage of attending more meetings in early recovery. In this respect, it may be helpful to keep in mind the advice commonly offered to AA newcomers: *attend ninety meetings in ninety days.*

Summing Up

Let's pause here to sum up what we've learned so far in part 2 from scientific research on the dynamics of AA: *how* it works. This will also summarize some ways to apply the information gleaned from the questions at the end of the previous chapters.

If we were to put these lessons from research in a nutshell, here is what they would teach someone who is contemplating turning to AA to help overcome an alcohol use disorder:

- *Work on changing your social network.* Consider moving away from friends and family whose own drinking— and attitudes about drinking—would tend to promote your drinking. If that does not seem feasible, then *add* some non-drinking friends to your social network.

- *Use AA as an alternative social network.* Don't simply go to meetings. Try on the idea of saying that you are a "member" of AA. See if you are comfortable with that being a part of your identity.

- *Get active in AA.* For example, make a few AA friends through meetings who you might call, email, text, or visit in person. Offer to do some service work like set-ting up a meeting or cleaning up afterward.

- *Seek out a temporary sponsor early.* Do not wait for some-one to volunteer to be your first temporary sponsor; instead, ask someone to do this for you. Your temporary sponsor may want you to stay in daily contact with him or her; if so, do that.

- *Explore the spiritual parts of AA.* This does not necessarily mean joining an organized religion or attending formal worship services. Rather, the spirituality that lies at the core of AA is about pursuing a life of meaning and values. These include honesty, the courage to admit to shortcomings, humility, and altruism. Within the AA culture these values are demonstrated through action.

By doing the above, the newcomer to AA will be following a prescription that has been laid out very clearly by the AA culture itself and confirmed through the thoughtful and carefully conducted studies we've reviewed here.

◆

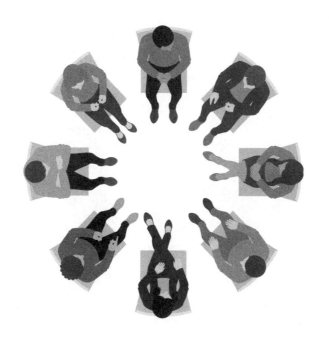

PART 3

Neurological Factors

Recovery and the Brain

In this chapter, I'd like to turn to an issue that is relevant to the topic of recovery, independent of whether that recovery is achieved through involvement in a Twelve Step program or some other means. That issue is how alcohol affects brain functioning and what happens to those effects if a person pursues abstinence.

It has long been established that chronic severe alcohol use can lead to irreversible neurological disorders including alcohol dementia, Wernicke's encephalopathy, and Korsakoff's syndrome. Typically, an acute case of encephalopathy or neurological damage (Wernicke's) precedes full-blown Korsakoff's, which is a form of dementia that is irreversible. The focus here is not on that end of the drinking spectrum and those consequences, but rather on the potential neurological consequences short of these disorders and whether those consequences are reversible in recovery.

Drinking and Brain Functioning

In a review of research on this subject, psychologists Jon Morgenstern and Marsha Bates of the Mount Sinai School of Medicine in New York reported that more than half of the individuals who enter treatment for alcohol or other substance use disorders have, at the outset, at least some impairment with respect to memory, tasks requiring new learning, or visual and perceptual skills (for example, completing mazes or playing simple computer games). What these researchers wanted to know was whether those deficits complicated treatment so as to render it less effective.

To answer their question, the researchers followed 118 individuals (70 men, 48 women) who entered treatment in two hospital-based treatment programs. To begin they administered a battery of neuropsychological tests to this group and found, again, that more than half showed at least some impairment. Specifically, 69 percent showed impairment on at least one of the seven tests that they took, 37 percent were impaired on two or more of the seven, and 14 percent on three or more. In short, the group demonstrated some degree of cognitive impairment at the outset of treatment, but it varied. Accordingly, they were divided into two groups:

- *Impaired:* Showing signs of cognitive impairment on at least two of seven tests

- *Non-impaired:* Showing signs of impairment on only one of seven tests

The treatment programs these men and women attended advocated AA attendance, though AA involvement, as defined in earlier chapters, was not their explicit goal. In addition, the participants were asked to respond to some questions aimed at measuring their affiliation with AA, as well as their commitment to abstinence as a personal goal. Finally, alcohol and drug use was assessed using a standard procedure in which the participants used a calendar to chart an estimate of their drinking or drug use on a daily basis over the past thirty days. This was reviewed at the end of treatment and again six months later.

The results of this study are significant as well as encouraging. Six months following treatment, both commitment to abstinence and AA affiliation were associated with dramatic decreases in alcohol and drug use. For example, six months post-treatment the percent of days when participants reported using alcohol or drugs was roughly 5 percent among those who indicated a strong commitment to abstinence. And the percent days abstinent was 95 percent among those who scored high on AA affiliation.

Now comes the surprise: contrary to expectations, Morgenstern and Bates *"found no support for the hypothesis that executive (neurological) impairment at treatment entry was a direct predictor of poorer drinking and other substance use outcomes 6 months following treatment."*

They also wrote that "the clinical significance of these findings would appear to be compelling." Indeed, they are. These findings are very encouraging, for they indicate that combining treatment with AA can be successful, even in the face of some neurological impairment at the outset. However, we need to keep in mind that these same results and conclusions might not apply to people with *severe* neurological impairments who seek treatment.

The longitudinal studies that we reviewed earlier, such as the sixteen-year study conducted by Moos and Moos (chapter 2), found that the best outcome for those seeking help for a drinking problem came from beginning AA and treatment simultaneously. If we assume that the men and women in the Moos study were comparable to the group studied by Morgenstern and Bates, then it's logical to assume that roughly half of them also suffered from some cognitive impairment due to drinking. Yet that did not impede their ability to recover.

Another thing to keep in mind in interpreting these findings is that they involve men and women who have been diagnosed with a substance use disorder. That means they are not low-risk drinkers—but neither are they all necessarily alcoholics. Still, about half of people within this range on the drinking spectrum can be expected to experience some neurological impairment. As noted earlier, these individuals may not attribute any such impairment to their drinking. They may, for instance, be experiencing some issues with memory or concentration that affect their lives in various ways, yet they may very well continue to drink at the same level and attribute these difficulties to other causes—age, stress, and so on. Mental health and medical professionals might be well advised, therefore, to query their clients not only about their drinking behavior, but also about any possible (perhaps subtle) neurological consequences.

In another study, researchers assessed brain functioning in 162 individuals who had been diagnosed as alcoholics (92 men and 70 women) and were in very early recovery (only three weeks sober), and compared that to a group of 165 non-alcoholics (83 men and 82 women). In the alcoholic group, 55 had been drinking between four and nine years; the remainder had been drinking between ten and thirty-three years. Obviously no one would describe this as a group of moderate drinkers. The researchers were specifically looking for evidence to support a belief—one that had been popular for a long time—that it takes about ten years of heavy drinking before the brain becomes affected by alcohol.

These researchers used select parts of a standard intelligence test to assess aspects of neuropsychological (brain) functioning such as memory, learning, and perceptual-motor coordination. What they found ran counter to the popular belief. First, both groups of alcoholics—those who had been drinking for ten years or more and those who had been drinking nine years or less—*did not differ significantly* from one another with respect to brain functioning.

Second, all of the diagnosed alcoholics in this study showed evidence of poorer brain functioning than the control group of non-alcoholics. It would appear, then, that heavy drinking (enough to qualify for a diagnosis of alcoholism) definitely interferes with brain functioning. However, that impairment also appears to occur relatively early on—at least for heavy drinkers—and then remains essentially unchanged for a long period of time.

Brain Functioning and Recovery

In 1996, Oscar Parsons and Sara Jo Nixon, who are affiliated with the Oklahoma Center for Alcohol and Drug-Related Studies, conducted a review of seventeen research studies on the cognitive functioning of people who drink. They were able to sort out these studies and report not only on the effects of drinking per se on brain functioning, but on degrees of drinking and how different degrees relate to cognitive functioning.

The studies included in this review included a wide range of tests on cognitive functioning. Some looked at the ability to make abstract comparisons (for example: *Hair is to humans as* _____ *are to fish*); others looked at the ability to solve math problems; still others assessed a person's ability to "translate" numbers into symbols or to put together puzzles. And so on. This diversity is actually good, since the collective findings might be more suspect if all the researchers chose identical measures.

Parsons and Nixon also grouped study participants according to how much alcohol they had consumed in the recent past (typically the past month). For example, one study of 1,201 men and women divided participants into the following categories: non-drinkers, very light drinkers, light drinkers, and moderate drinkers. In this case *moderate drinking* was defined as consuming no more than three drinks per day. Another study included the following groups: non-drinkers, social drinkers, alcoholics, and abstinent alcoholics. Here *social* meant consuming ninety or fewer drinks a month—a lot!

The fact that different studies defined their groups differently is not an issue, as Parsons and Nixon were able to fold them all into their own categories. Here is what they concluded:

- People drinking five to six alcoholic drinks per day over an extended period of time show some neurological effects, as measured by the various tests cited above.

- At seven to ten drinks per day, mild neurological effects become apparent.

- At ten or more drinks per day over a prolonged period of time, moderate effects on brain functioning are present.

In their review, these researchers also make a point of stating that, among women as compared to men, the above numbers should probably be reduced by one or two drinks per day. This makes sense, given the differences in the way women and men metabolize alcohol. In addition, when they further divided the seventeen studies into those that focused on people with an average age of thirty-two or younger compared to those with an average age of thirty-three and older, they found no differences. In other words, they found a direct connection between how much people drink on a regular basis and alcohol's effects on the brain—and this was as true for older people as it was for younger people. Thus, any belief that young people are somehow immune to the physical (in this case, neurological) effects of alcohol would appear to be a myth.

Thus far in this chapter we have been able to reach several conclusions about the brain and recovery. First, we know that roughly half of people who seek formal treatment for a drinking problem (and also perhaps as many who just opt for AA) will have some brain impairment at that starting point. That impairment is linked to their drinking, and its severity will vary depending on how much and how long they've been drinking. Being younger gives a person no advantage in this area; however, being female means that impaired brain function will be worse than for a male given comparable drinking histories.

Now for the upside: that brain impairment (assuming it is not truly severe) does not appear to stand as a barrier to recovery.

Oscar Parsons, co-author of the above study, was a leader in research investigating the effects of alcohol on brain functioning for several decades. In 1997, he was the recipient of the Distinguished Research Award of the Research Social on Alcoholism.

In one of Parsons's last publications he again raised this issue of whether deficits in brain functioning might exist on a continuum, or spectrum—much like the idea that "the drinking world," as we discussed earlier (chapter 4), exists on a spectrum. In that paper he pointed out that he, his students, and his colleagues had for twenty-five years studied the effects of alcohol abuse on "information processing, cognitive, perceptual, and perceptual-motor functions of the human brain"—in short, on key aspects of brain functioning.

Parsons first organized and then summarized the results of

many studies of alcohol and brain functioning among men and women whose brain impairments ranged from most severe (Korsakoff's syndrome) to those associated with a drinking spectrum that ran from heavy to moderate to light. One question he sought to answer has a great meaning to men and women who choose abstinence and recovery as their solution for an alcohol use disorder: if the recovering alcoholic remains sober, is there remission of neurocognitive deficits, and if so, how long does it take?

The studies conducted by the Oklahoma group, along with others included in Parsons's review, were consistent with the "spectrum hypothesis"; that is, the severity of cognitive deficits from drinking correlates with both how much and how long a person drinks, with *heavy drinking* defined as more than twenty-one drinks per week. Note, however, that this level of drinking still does not necessarily qualify for a diagnosis of severe alcohol disorder (alcoholism).

A major study conducted by this research center assessed brain functioning in two groups of alcoholics: one that had been sober for one month, and another that had been sober for four years. They also compared these groups to a third group of non-alcoholics. What they found was that brain functioning in the group with only one month of sobriety showed significant deficits. In contrast, among those in the long-term sobriety group, "for practical purposes they had recovered to near normal levels of performance."

To summarize, it appears that brain functioning can recover, too, as part of overall recovery from an alcohol use disorder. However, brain functioning takes time to recover, perhaps even years. Despite that slow process of recovery, as demonstrated by studies we reviewed earlier, impaired cognitive functioning does not, in and of itself, appear to present a barrier to recovery; rather, its healing is an added benefit of recovery.

One last study of brain functioning and recovery that we'll review was conducted by Neurological Research, Inc., in Corte Madera, California, by a team lead by George Fein, PhD. They recruited 91 men and women (42 of them women), with an average age of sixty-seven, through postings at AA meetings in the San Francisco Bay area. They targeted this population because they wanted to assess brain functioning in people with alcohol use disorders who were now abstinent. Indeed, the men and women in this group had been abstinent from alcohol for an average of nearly fifteen years.

Fein and his co-researcher, Shannon McGillivray, further divided their sample into three subgroups:

people who started abstaining from alcohol before age fifty

those who began their recovery between age fifty and sixty

individuals who began their recovery after age sixty

For a comparison group, Fein and McGillivray recruited 22 men and 30 women with an average age of sixty-eight who had a lifetime drinking average of less than thirty drinks per month and who had never had more than sixty drinks in one month.

To assess their brain functioning, all participants were given a battery of tests too extensive to list here. Suffice it to say these tests either included or complemented those used in standard intelligence assessments as well as tests designed to assess cognitive functioning in individuals with brain damage. These tests all include normative data so it's possible to tell whether an individual (or group) falls below average on any of them—thereby indicating less-than-normal brain functioning. In addition, they assessed a comparison group of 52 men and women of a similar age who had never had an alcohol use disorder.

Here is what these researchers found, in their own words:

> Overall, the elderly abstinent groups performed comparably to controls on the assessment of cognitive function. . . . Our data show that elderly alcoholics that drank late into life, but with at least 6 months of abstinence can exhibit normal cognitive functioning.

At first blush the above results might seem like cause for celebration. They do show that, for at least some elderly recovering alcoholics, it is possible to recover brain functioning as long as they remain abstinent for a minimum of six months. However, it could be dangerous to assume that these results apply to all men and women who drink heavily relatively late into life and who then stop. In particular, do these findings imply that it's okay to drink heavily up until you are in your sixties, and then have normal brain functioning after stopping for just six months? Not necessarily. Why? One reason might be that the individuals who agreed to participate in this brain functioning study were not truly representative of all elderly alcoholics—even those who are in recovery. They may, rather, be representative of a group of older men and women who have been in recovery on average for some time, but who as a group are also healthier and more robust than average. In this *selective survivorship* scenario, healthier alcoholics may be more likely to live into their sixties, seventies, and eighties, and as a result perform better on these tests of brain functioning. With that in mind, it may be significant to note that the group of recovering elderly men and women had on average larger craniums than the men and women in the non-alcoholic comparison group. It's possible that this difference translated in more "reserve capacity" in their brains (like a reserve gas tank!) and that this reserve capacity is what allowed them to recover their brain functioning so well.

Even with the above cautionary note in mind, it is still encouraging to know that the brain appears to be a fairly resilient organ, one that is capable of bouncing back, as it were, even later in life.

Summing Up

The research reviewed in this chapter strongly supports the idea that the brain can recover from alcohol use, even heavy and chronic alcohol use. To be sure, there are cases where brain damage from chronic alcoholism may be irreversible, as in cases of alcohol dementia associated with Korsakoff's syndrome. However, these appear to be the exception as opposed to the rule.

Alcohol abuse definitely does have negative effects on brain function. Research by Parsons and his colleagues suggests that these effects are not black-and-white (something you either have or don't have, period), but instead exist on a spectrum that mirrors the range of drinking from low risk through a zone that includes mild and moderate use to severe use or alcoholism at the other extreme. Negative effects on cognitive functioning may begin to appear anywhere along this spectrum and can be expected to get worse as a drinking problem intensifies.

Half of the men and women who enter a treatment program for drinking already have some evidence of brain impairment. It's reasonable to assume that a comparable number of people may be impaired when they finally decide to try AA and abstinence as a solution. Significantly, this brain impairment does not seem to stop many of these individuals from pursuing treatment, AA, or both. By the same token, we cannot be certain whether or not brain dysfunction is actually a barrier to treatment and recovery for some.

The studies we've looked at here all focused on the brains of individuals who were abstinent from alcohol use for some period of time. We don't know what the outcomes would be for people who chose to continue drinking moderately. However, because several studies have showed a connection between cognitive dysfunction and even moderate drinking, we know that brain function may very well continue to be affected if a person continues to drink at more than a low-risk level. Moreover, these individuals may not attribute subtle neurological deficits to their drinking.

For those who pursue abstinence as opposed to reduced drinking, brain recovery begins quickly and improves steadily. Complete recovery appears possible, though it may take years. That brain recovery, however, is then correlated with all the other benefits of recovery, with respect to mental health, spiritual development, and so on. Taken together, the physical, spiritual, social, and mental health manifestations of recovery may constitute the "promise" that is often spoken of in AA.

◆

Mental Illness and Twelve Step Recovery

A significant number of men and women who have an alcohol use disorder also suffer from some form of mental illness. These can range from depression, anxiety, and post-traumatic stress disorder to bipolar disorder and even schizophrenia.

To put this in context, we need to look back on the way that drinking problems were defined in chapter 4. There I presented the notion that the "drinking world" could be represented by a spectrum that runs from low-risk drinking at one end to a severe alcohol use disorder at the other. Between these two extremes are many "shades of gray" that correspond to how much and how often a person drinks. One area along this continuum has been labeled in the American Psychiatric Association's new *Diagnostic and Statistical Manual of Mental Disorders* (5th ed.; *DSM-5*) as a *mild* alcohol use disorder, and another has been labeled a *moderate* alcohol use disorder. With this in mind, let's look at some of the data that has been collected on the relationship between drinking and mental illness.

Alcohol Use and Its Relation to Mental Illness

The National Institute on Alcohol Abuse and Alcoholism (NIAAA) funded a national survey regarding alcohol use and its relation to mental illness. The survey was designed to reflect the entire U.S. population, and data were collected through interviews. In all, 20,291 people ages eighteen and older were interviewed. The interview was intended to collect information about the participants' experiences during the previous year. Confidentiality was guaranteed so as to facilitate getting accurate information.

This survey focused primarily on men and women whose drinking fell into one of two zones on the drinking spectrum: moderate alcohol use disorders and severe alcohol use disorders. To collect data representative of the entire population, the researchers also interviewed men and women who had neither a significant drinking problem nor a mental illness. In the interviews, subjects were asked how much they drank and whether they had ever been diagnosed with one of a number of psychiatric illnesses. Rather than trying to determine whether the individuals being interviewed were in treatment for either a drinking problem or a mental illness, the researchers wanted to learn how many people had

- *both* a mental illness and a substance use disorder (dual diagnoses, or co-occurring disorders)
- *either* a mental illness or a substance use disorder
- *neither* a mental illness nor a substance use disorder

Let's take a look at what this research yielded. The authors not only reported simple percentages, but also presented their data in a unique way: in terms of the odds of having a particular mental illness if your drinking pattern fell into either a moderate or severe category, as opposed to not having these drinking problems. Here is what they found:

Mental Illness	Odds _Moderate Alcohol Disorder_	Odds _Severe Alcohol Disorder_
Depression	1.1 to 1	3.9 to 1
Anxiety	1.7 to 1	2.6 to 1
PTSD	1.5 to 1	2.2 to 1
Schizophrenia	1.9 to 1	3.8 to 1

What can we conclude from the data in this table? It tells us, for example, that men and women whose drinking places them at the moderate alcohol use disorder zone on the drinking spectrum and people who have no alcohol use disorder have about equal chances of having suffered from depression in the previous year (a 1.1 to 1 ratio). In other words, this level of drinking does not appear to pose a greater risk than average for depression.

On the other hand, men and women with a severe drinking problem are almost four times as likely to have experienced depression in the previous year compared with people who have no drinking problem (a 3.9 to 1 ratio).

As for anxiety disorders and post-traumatic stress disorder (PTSD), there is a direct relationship between where someone is on the drinking spectrum and the likelihood that he or she has one of these disorders. For example, the 1.7 to 1 ratio for anxiety disorders means that people with a moderate alcohol use disorder are 70 percent more likely to suffer from an anxiety disorder than those whose drinking pattern falls somewhere short of that. And if they move into the severe alcohol use disorder zone, they are more than twice as likely to have an anxiety disorder than people who drink less.

With PTSD, we see once more a relationship between drinking and that disorder, such that heavier drinkers are more likely than people without a drinking problem to suffer from this often debilitating disorder.

The same is true to an even greater extent for the diagnosis of schizophrenia: the heavy drinker is much more likely to have that additional diagnosis.

So what does this all mean? Does it indicate that drinking *causes* anxiety, depression, PTSD, and even schizophrenia? Probably not, as it does not make sense that drinking by itself could cause such a diverse range of mental illnesses. What it does suggest, however, are several things:

- A significant number (though by no means all) of men and women who seek treatment for a drinking problem, or decide to go to AA for that reason, suffer from some form of mental illness *in addition to* their drinking problem.

- People with more severe drinking problems (alcoholism) are even more likely to have an additional mental illness. It is possible that their drinking has made their mental illness worse, or alternatively, that they have turned to drinking as a means of self-medicating their mental illness.

- The best approach to helping these individuals would be to recognize the existence of this dual diagnosis, or co-occurring disorder, and treat both the mental illness and the drinking problem *at the same time.*

The idea that some people who end up with a significant drinking problem may have first turned to alcohol to relieve symptoms of a mental illness is worth a further look. It's well known, for example, that men and women who suffer from PTSD—such as soldiers exposed to chronic stress as a result of multiple deployments to combat zones—also abuse alcohol and other drugs, especially cannabis. They may indeed have used alcohol (or cannabis) to relieve symptoms such as anxiety, edginess, poor sleep, and even flashbacks.

A question that is relevant to this book relates to how AA itself may affect mental illnesses such as depression or even PTSD. In other words, could it be that getting *involved* in AA, as that term has been defined here, can itself help ameliorate some of the symptoms associated with a mental illness such as depression or PTSD? This is a question we'll look at shortly.

Further Data on the Dually Diagnosed

George Fein is a researcher whose work in the area of brain dysfunction was mentioned in the last chapter. In another study, Fein looked into the prevalence of psychiatric diagnoses in recovering alcoholics. To do this he recruited 293 individuals in the Honolulu area through postings at AA meetings. He divided this group into those men and women who reported being abstinent between five and fifteen weeks, which he called the short-term abstinent (STA) group, and a group who reported being abstinent between one and a half and thirty-two years. This group was designated the long-term abstinent (LTA) group.

Next, Fein assessed all the participants for psychiatric disorders. To do this, he used a measure, which is administered in a one-to-one interview format, that yields information on whether an individual has no psychiatric diagnosis versus having had one of the following diagnoses *at some point* in his or her life:

- bipolar disorder
- dysthymia (chronic low-grade depression)
- major depression
- agoraphobia (anxiety associated with being in open spaces)
- panic disorder (anxiety associated with panic attacks)
- post-traumatic stress disorder (which includes symptoms of both depression and anxiety)
- social phobia (anxiety associated with interpersonal interactions)

What Fein discovered was fairly dramatic. First, more than 60 percent of the individuals in *either* the STA or the LTA groups reported having received a diagnosis associated with either anxiety or depression (so-called mood disorders) at some point in their lives. This compared to just 15 percent among a control group of non-alcohol abusing men and women. This confirms the data reported above—that men and women with severe (and perhaps even moderate) drinking problems are likely to also have had a psychiatric diagnosis at some point.

Equally important is Fein's finding that there were no differences between the group that had been sober for only a few weeks and those who had been sober from a year and a half to as long as thirty-two years. In Fein's own words, "Such diagnoses do not impact one's ability to achieve or maintain abstinence." That's not to say that diagnoses such as anxiety or depression could not benefit from treatment. What it means, though, is that these mental illnesses, much like the mild to moderate brain impairment that we looked at in the last chapter, do not appear to constitute a major barrier to recovery.

Involvement in AA or NA within the Dual Diagnosis Population
We know, then, from rigorous surveys like the above that a significant proportion of men and women who have moderate or severe drinking problems also have a mental illness. One thing we would also want to know about this population is how it compares to the population of men and women who have only a substance use disorder, particularly with respect to whether they turn to Twelve Step fellowships like AA and NA for help.

A study reported in the journal *Psychiatric Services* offers a window into this issue. The researchers divided men and women who sought treatment in a hospital setting into two groups: those who had *only* a substance use disorder and those who were dually diagnosed with *both* a substance use disorder and a mental illness. The total group numbered 351, and they were followed to see whether they utilized AA or NA after leaving treatment.

The results of this study are encouraging, for the researchers found comparable rates of attendance at AA or NA for the two groups, with the notable exception of men and women who were diagnosed as schizophrenic. AA/NA attendance among this latter group was significantly lower. If looked at from the perspective of diagnosis, this result makes sense. It also points to a direction and a goal for those who treat schizophrenics with co-occurring alcohol use disorders. Schizophrenia itself is associated with impaired social skills—the very skills required to become active in a Twelve Step fellowship. It is therefore understandable that this group would have a harder time getting active in AA or NA. With that in mind, clinicians would do well to recognize this challenge and work toward enhancing the social skills and reducing social anxiety within this group of people as much as possible.

Despite the results for this one dually diagnosed group, this survey affirms again that having a mental illness in and of itself need not pose a barrier to utilizing Twelve Step programs. However, in fairness, these individuals should be aware that there was a time when Twelve Step fellowships were not so welcoming of the dually diagnosed. Some individuals have shared with me that they were told that they should not attend AA because they were "using drugs," referring in this case to prescription medications for mental illness. And a few substance abuse counselors who themselves are dually diagnosed have said that they believe some people who go to AA for their recovery choose not to disclose their mental illness for fear of being rejected.

This situation has given rise to several Twelve Step recovery groups for people with co-occurring psychiatric and substance use disorders. One of them, Double Trouble in Recovery (DTR), has several hundred groups around the country and a number of research studies have been published showing its effectiveness. The second most prevalent group nationally, Dual Recovery Anonymous (DRA), similarly, has its own literature and website. The newest group, Dual Diagnosis Anonymous (DDA), is mainly concentrated in Oregon but is well organized and has plans to grow. All of these groups accept people with mental illness no matter how severe, and they encourage members to talk about their struggles with their psychiatric symptoms and medications as well as their substance use.

What Does AA Have to Say about Psychiatric Medications?

As we know, AA itself does not dictate "policy." However, AA members often speak out—rendering opinions as opposed to policy. In that vein a group of physicians who are also AA members and identified only as "friends of AA" collaborated to write the pamphlet mentioned earlier, *The AA Member—Medications and Other Drugs.* This document, directed to recovering individuals as well as to medical professionals, addresses the issue of medication use (and misuse) straightforwardly. It acknowledges first that "some AA members must take prescribed medication for serious medical problems." It then adds a caveat: "It is generally accepted that the *misuse* of prescription medication and other drugs can threaten the achievement and maintenance of sobriety."

This pamphlet, modeling the Big Book, includes first-person accounts from men and women who needed to address both their mental illness and their alcohol use disorder if they had any hope for recovery. Here is an example:

> Each time I abruptly stopped taking my medication
> my symptoms got worse and my suicidal depression
> came back.

The bottom line, then, is that individuals who are dually diagnosed do appear to utilize Twelve Step fellowships, and that at least some AA members (as represented by the above "friends of AA") support the responsible use of medications through an open and informed patient-doctor relationship.

Other Medications: Anti-craving Drugs

Though anti-craving medications are not in any way part of the AA Twelve Step model of recovery, the reality is that many practitioners and clinics now incorporate these medications into their treatment programs—even those that also advocate for AA. The National Association of State Alcohol and Drug Abuse Directors, which issued a brief on this subject in 2001, noted the increase in the use of medications of all sorts, ranging from anti-craving drugs to anti-depressants, as adjuncts to treatment. What do we know about how the use of these drugs interacts with Twelve Step recovery?

In a study involving 70 men diagnosed as alcohol dependent, Joseph Volpicelli and colleagues studied the effects of naltrexone, which is intended to stop alcohol cravings, versus a placebo. This was a "double-blind" study, so the volunteers did not know whether they had been given the medication or a placebo and neither did those who monitored them. The researchers found that, indeed, those men who received the anti-craving medication reported fewer cravings over the twelve-week period in which they took the medication as compared to the group who received a placebo. The most dramatic effects were seen among those men who had a slip while in treatment. Half of those who received the naltrexone reported a full relapse after such a slip. While a 50 percent relapse rate may seem high, it doesn't compare to the experience of the placebo group: of the twenty men taking the placebo who slipped, nineteen went on to have a full relapse.

Though the use of naltrexone may help to reduce cravings, what is notably lacking from studies like the above is *what kind of treatment* the men were receiving. As we've seen from our review of research, this matters a lot.

A team of researchers led by Stephanie O'Malley, PhD, at the Yale University School of Medicine took another look at the effects of the anti-craving drug naltrexone. They followed a group of 97 men who were alcohol dependent and who were also prescribed either a placebo or naltrexone, and assessed them six months after treatment. Two treatments were involved but neither was Twelve Step focused. One was a coping skills therapy similar to the CBT described earlier; the other was a vaguely described "supportive therapy." The men received naltrexone through twelve weeks of one of these treatments, at which point the medication (along with counseling) was discontinued.

This study, then, may not be relevant when it comes to looking at the evidence in support of AA and Twelve Step-focused treatments. On the other hand, one result is instructive. O'Malley and her team found that "the effect of naltrexone therapy on abstinence rates persisted only through the first month of follow-up." So although the anti-craving medication may have helped reduce cravings, the effect was relatively short-lived once it was terminated.

Another anti-craving medication that is seeing increased use is actually a combination of two drugs, buprenorphine and naloxone. It is used to reduce cravings for opioids, including heroin and prescription pain medications. A multisite study of the use of buprenorphine/naloxone, led by Roger Weiss, MD, of McLean Hospital and Harvard Medical School, assessed the effectiveness of that drug on 653 individuals (38 percent women) who had been diagnosed as dependent on prescription opioids. These individuals also received counseling.

The results of this study, with opioids as opposed to alcohol, largely mirror those reported by O'Malley, specifically the conclusion: If tapered off buprenorphine-naloxone, even after 12 weeks of treatment, the likelihood of an unsuccessful outcome is high, even in patients receiving counseling.

So what can we say at this point about the use of anti-craving medications as treatments for addiction? It appears that two things are true: First, these drugs do seem to have the power to reduce cravings. Second, these medications alone are not sufficient to achieve long-term recovery. With that in mind, it is important to also acknowledge the limitations of short-term treatments for substance use disorders. They, much like these anti-craving medications, may fade easily. In contrast, we know from all we've reviewed here that it is *sustained* involvement in a Twelve Step fellowship that is associated with long-term recovery.

A Research Study with Dually Diagnosed Young Adults

One study looked at Twelve Step fellowship participation and involvement of a group of young adults who were diagnosed with both an alcohol use disorder and a mental illness. This collaborative study involved researchers at the Center for Addiction Medicine at Massachusetts General Hospital, Harvard Medical School, and the Hazelden Foundation in Minnesota. The participants were young adults (74 percent of them men) between the ages of eighteen and twenty-four who attended a residential treatment program for young people with substance use disorders; some also had mental health diagnoses.

The dual diagnosis (DD) group represented 47 percent of these young adults entering treatment; 53 percent had a substance use disorder only (SUD). For the DD group, primary diagnoses included mood disorders such as depression, dysthymia, anxiety disorder, social phobia, and panic disorder. These diagnoses essentially mirror those of the subjects in Fein's study of adults in recovery. The 47 percent figure (representing those with a dual diagnosis of substance use disorder and mental illness) is also consistent with other findings.

This group received treatment that was based in the Twelve Step model and which included Twelve Step Facilitation (TSF), which, as we learned in chapter 3, emphasizes AA attendance and involvement. For this project, that involvement was measured using an instrument that assessed meeting participation (speaking), fellowship involvement (contact with a sponsor), and Step work (progress in working through the Twelve Step program). In addition, the total number of AA meetings attended was tracked. As you can see, this assessment has to do with "working it," not just "being there" when it comes to Twelve Step recovery.

Treatment outcome (recovery) was measured using a statistic that we are familiar with: the percentage of days that an individual is abstinent (PDA), along with a measure of alcohol and drug use: the Inventory of Drug Use Consequences. The latter was used because among this group of young adults (indeed, as is increasingly true universally), it is not simply alcohol abuse but polysubstance abuse that is the more accurate substance abuse diagnosis.

This group was assessed at three, six, and again at twelve months after completing treatment. It was found, first, that both those young people in the dual diagnosis (DD) group and those in the substance use disorder only (SUD) groups attended AA or NA meetings at about the same rate.

At three months post-treatment, both groups were *attending* meetings on roughly 50 percent of days. By six months this had tapered off to about 40 percent of days, and at the twelve-month mark it was 30 percent of the time. Despite that drop-off in meeting attendance, these young adults were still going to meetings a good percentage of the time.

As measured by Twelve Step fellowship involvement, both groups maintained a steady and significant level of involvement after completing treatment. In other words, collectively their scores on the involvement scale were high following treatment and remained so even twelve months later.

So, what about recovery? How did these two groups fare? Well, to begin, both attendance and involvement were linked with better outcomes—meaning more days without drinking. We've seen this result before, of course, but in science another replication never hurts. Here, using a new group of individuals, and using a new measure of Twelve Step involvement, we see once more that "working it" is strongly predictive of recovery.

Despite their similarities with respect to attendance and involvement, the DD group as a whole had fewer percent days abstinent than the SUD group. That's not to say that treatment failed for the DD group; on the contrary, greater involvement was still associated with better recovery for this group. And for the DD group one factor in particular—having a sponsor—stood out as a predictor of recovery. Nevertheless, the DD group did not fare quite as well as the SUD group.

So what advice would we offer to someone who has a mental illness—such as depression, anxiety, or PTSD—and also needs to pursue recovery from a substance use disorder? First, we know from the studies cited above that their mental illness need not be a barrier to recovery. Many men and women with long-term recovery have suffered from a mental illness at some point in their lives. Second, we would want to point out (yet again) one component of involvement that may make the biggest difference to their recovery: get a sponsor, and get one early! Also, the individual with a severe mental illness might try one of the Twelve Step dual recovery groups mentioned above. A major drawback with these groups is that they can be hard to find and, unlike AA and NA, aren't yet available in many areas. (Note: If you can't find one of these meetings, you can still attend AA or NA. Although the talk in AA and NA meetings is usually restricted to staying clean and sober, and so you will have limited opportunity to share information about your mental illness in that context, you may very well find a sponsor and other group members who are also dealing with both a substance use disorder and a mental illness.)

Specific Mental Illnesses and Twelve Step Recovery

In recent years researchers have begun to delve more deeply into the dual diagnosis phenomenon. In particular, they have been interested in determining whether there is a relationship between Twelve Step recovery and specific mental illnesses—in other words, might they interact in any way? As I write this book, this area of study is relatively new, and though initial findings are promising, we still have much to learn, in particular about how involvement in a Twelve Step program might affect a mental illness. In this section we'll look at studies regarding two of the most common disorders, depression and PTSD.

Depression

The first series of studies we'll discuss were conducted under the leadership of Sandra A. Brown, a professor of psychiatry and psychology at the University of California–San Diego. The study participants were men and women who had been diagnosed with both a substance use disorder (alcohol and/or drugs) and major depression. These studies compared two different approaches to treating this dual diagnosis combination. One was integrated cognitive behavioral therapy, or ICBT. This approach, much like the CBT described earlier, seeks primarily to teach coping skills and other strategies to relieve depression and help people reduce and resist alcohol or other drug use. ICBT is a manual-guided treatment that is broken down into three broad components:

- *Education:* Educating the patient about the nature of depression and how it is affected by substance abuse
- *Mindfulness meditation:* Teaching the patient specific techniques for relaxing and stress reduction
- *Cognitive restructuring:* Helping the patient understand how thoughts and emotions interact in specific situations to result in certain actions; and then to help restructure these connections to alter emotional reactions and behavior (such as drinking)

The second treatment was Twelve Step Facilitation (TSF), which, as we learned in chapter 3, is a manual-guided treatment whose goal is not simply to encourage Twelve Step meeting attendance, but to systematically educate and coach people with substance use disorders to participate in a Twelve Step fellowship.

Participants in both ICBT and TSF received standard pharmacological treatment—antidepressants—in addition to these interventions. In each of these studies, ICBT was expected to be superior to TSF, since it was designed to target depression specifically, whereas TSF is aimed at the substance use disorder half of the dual diagnosis.

In their first study, 66 military veterans (61 of them men) diagnosed with both major depression and a substance use disorder were recruited from the Veterans Administration San Diego Healthcare System. They were randomly assigned to either ICBT of TSF, and both their substance use and their depression were assessed at four points in time: midway through treatment, at the end of treatment, three months post-treatment, and six months post-treatment.

The findings of this study were complex and enlightening—all that you can expect from research. First, the depression scores among study participants receiving TSF actually decreased more than the scores among the ICBT group during active treatment. Then, three months after treatment, the groups were equal on depression but still lower than when they began treatment. But at the six-month mark, depression had returned to roughly its starting level among the TSF group, whereas it rose only slightly in the ICBT group.

As for Twelve Step involvement and substance use, this relationship was once more confirmed: greater Twelve Step involvement was associated with higher percent days abstinent. At the midway point in treatment, the TSF group had slightly higher average PDA scores (95 percent) than the ICBT group (90 percent). In this regard, we should note that the men and women who received ICBT were free to attend AA meetings, and they did so nearly as often as those who received TSF, which may account for the small difference. As was true for depression, though, this effect seemed to dissipate over time for the TSF group—though it never went as low as it had been prior to treatment—to the point where the TSF reported being abstinent a little more than 70 percent of the time, as compared to more than 80 percent of the time for the ICBT group.

So what might account for the above trends? One possibility is that the techniques that the ICBT group learned tended to stick with them over time, while whatever healing powers came from Twelve Step involvement did not. There is some evidence for this conclusion. For example, one study involving a group of individuals with both depression and substance use disorders reported less AA involvement—they were less likely to have an AA sponsor, they had fewer AA friends, and they reported less contact with those friends—following treatment as compared to a group that had only a substance use disorder (no depression).

In effect, the dual-diagnosis group was less involved in the Twelve Step fellowship (as we've defined it here) than the group with only the substance use disorder. It could well be that this "dilution" in AA involvement was related to the loss of those positive effects that occurred with TSF during active treatment.

In another study conducted by this same group, 209 subjects who had both an alcohol use disorder and depression were recruited through the Veterans Administration health care system. They were randomly assigned to either ICBT or TSF, and they were assessed at three, six, and nine months after treatment. As in the previous study, these individuals also received medication for their depression.

The researchers again predicted that the ICBT treatment would be superior to TSF since it was specifically designed to address both depression and substance abuse using cognitive behavioral interventions whereas TSF's single goal is Twelve Step fellowship involvement as a means of facilitating recovery. They measured depression as well as monitoring drinking days and drinks per drinking day.

The results of this second study build upon and also add to those from the smaller initial study. Here is a summary of the findings:

- Greater Twelve Step meeting attendance and greater Twelve Step fellowship involvement predicted both lower depression and less substance use.

- TSF led to significantly lower levels of depression during active treatment as compared to ICBT.

- The positive effect of TSF on depression came directly as a result of meeting attendance, accounting for nearly a quarter of that effect.

- Lower depression scores at the three- and six-month follow-ups predicted lower drinking at months six and nine. That is, less drinking was associated with less depression.

This study ends with the following conclusion:

> For patients with substance dependence and major depressive disorder, attendance at 12 step meetings is associated with mental health benefits that extend beyond substance use, and reduced depression could be a key mechanism whereby 12 step meetings reduce future drinking in this population.

What these researchers are suggesting is extraordinary. In effect, they are saying that recovery from alcoholism and addiction through active participation in a Twelve Step fellowship can be part of a "cure" for depression, and that cure in turn facilitates further recovery from both a substance use disorder and a mental illness.

These findings should not in any way be taken as a criticism of ICBT or the skills it teaches. On the contrary, ICBT is an effective treatment. There is no good reason for competition between these two treatment modes. In fact, combining the two, as many clinicians do now (many include motivational enhancement therapy as well), might best serve individuals dually diagnosed with depression and a substance use disorder.

We can take away one other lesson from these two studies, and that has to do with potential "deterioration" in AA involvement among people who suffer from depression. It appears that TSF as a treatment was quite effective in boosting AA attendance and involvement, and in turn at reducing both substance use and depression. However, it is what happens to that attendance and involvement, say a year after treatment, that can be critical to continued recovery from both mental illness and substance abuse. In that case, maintaining AA involvement needs to be the focus of treatment.

This same theme of the possible palliative effects of Twelve Step involvement on mental illness was also picked up on by researchers at the Massachusetts General Hospital and Harvard Medical School. They employed sophisticated statistical techniques to analyze the results of a study of 1,706 adults who had been diagnosed with severe alcohol use disorders (alcoholism). To measure depression these men and women completed the Beck Depression Inventory. This is an established measure of depression that inquires about a person's mood, energy level, and so on—all symptoms of depression—and yields scores ranging from 0 to 63, with higher scores indicating more severe depression. The researchers also measured AA meeting attendance and alcohol use, and then assessed these men and women for alcohol use, AA attendance, and depression following treatment. Here is what they found: greater AA attendance was associated with better alcohol use outcomes and decreased depression.

The researchers similarly concluded:

> AA appears to lead both to improvements in alcohol use and psychological and emotional wellbeing, which in turn may reinforce further abstinence and recovery-related change.

The research we've reviewed in earlier chapters certainly supports the idea that recovery leads to steady improvements in a person's overall health and quality of life. These researchers' collective assertion, then—that recovery from addiction also facilitates recovery from depression—makes a lot of sense.

Twelve Step Recovery and PTSD

A second dually diagnosed population that has been the subject of research are those who suffer from post-traumatic stress disorder, or PTSD. The study we will examine here was spearheaded by Elisa Triffleman, MD, who at the time of the research was affiliated with the Department of Psychiatry at Yale University School of Medicine. Her study compared two different approaches to treating PTSD and was reported in the journal *Alcoholism Treatment Quarterly.*

The participants in this study were nine men and ten women who all had been diagnosed with both PTSD and substance dependence (severe substance use disorders involving alcohol or other drugs). They were each randomly assigned to one of two treatments:

- *Substance Dependence Post-Traumatic-Stress-Disorder Therapy (SDPT):* This treatment was the one that Triffleman and her co-investigators devised and then predicted would be the more successful of the two treatments tested. SDPT, similar to the ICBT model discussed in the previous section, is a cognitive behavioral treatment that includes components such as Stress Inoculation Therapy, systematic desensitization, and *in vivo* exposure therapy. Systematic desensitization seeks to teach clients with PTSD first to relax and then to imagine a stressful event related to their PTSD, the idea being that this will help to reduce symptoms such as anxiety. Stress inoculation and in vivo exposure work in a similar fashion, although in the in vivo variation the client is exposed to a real-life situation that resembles an actual traumatic event as closely as possible. All of these interventions were incorporated into a single therapeutic package. Men and women assigned to SDPT completed an average of twenty-six individual therapy sessions.

- *Twelve Step Facilitation Therapy (TSF):* As we know, TSF facilitates active involvement (or what has been called *categorical* involvement) in a Twelve Step fellowship. According to the researchers in this study, TSF was intended to serve as a control treatment. In other words it was a treatment that was not expected to yield good results as compared to SDPT. The men and women assigned to TSF completed an average of sixteen individual therapy sessions.

The authors listed the following central hypotheses for this clinical trial:

- Treatment with SDPT would result in large decreases in substance abuse severity as compared to TSF
- Treatment with SDPT would lead to substantial decreases in PTSD symptoms and severity, and improvement on measures of overall mental health as compared to TSF

It did not turn out that way. Here are the results as reported:

Other than for the SDPT participants receiving more therapy sessions than the TSF participants there were no significant differences in outcomes between treatments. In the sample as a whole there was improvement on measures of substance abuse, PTSD severity, and psychiatric severity.

What is most striking to me about these results is not that SDPT and TSF both worked, but that once again a treatment aimed at involving participants in a Twelve Step fellowship would be as effective at reducing symptoms of PTSD as a treatment designed specifically to do this. The implication repeats itself and is clear: *active involvement and commitment to a Twelve Step fellowship has healing powers beyond recovery from substance use disorders.*

As was true for the studies that employed integrated cognitive behavioral therapy, this conclusion about the palliative effects of being involved in a Twelve Step program does not mean that people diagnosed with PTSD should not also be involved in treatments like SDPT. Indeed, research is showing the effectiveness of PTSD treatments that incorporate elements such as gradual exposure to traumatic memories and meditation techniques. At the same time these results on Twelve Step recovery and mental illness, while early, show the potential value of using a two-pronged approach that combines TSF with treatments like SDPT, especially for people diagnosed with both PTSD and a substance use disorder.

Substance Abuse: Symptom or Illness?

Results such as the ones we've examined here, on the healing power of Twelve Step recovery on mental illness, can shed some light on a long-standing debate within the mental health community. That debate centers on the very nature of substance use disorders—specifically, whether they are essentially *symptoms* of other mental illnesses or are independent.

Those who favor the former view have been inclined to believe that a substance use disorder would "spontaneously remit" (disappear) once the underlying mental illness was treated. In other words, if alcohol or other substance use disorders are a side effect of depression (or PTSD), then they should go away once the depression (or PTSD) is treated. Yet the results we've seen in this chapter point to exactly the opposite conclusion: that treating a substance use disorder through active involvement in a Twelve Step fellowship can actually help to heal mental illnesses such as depression and PTSD.

Summing Up

Research into the connection between recovery from substance use disorders and mental health has only begun, but the findings reported here suggest that recovery itself—and in particular Twelve Step recovery—has healing powers of its own. Nonetheless, many questions remain. For example, what components of Twelve Step recovery are the most powerful in relieving mental illness? Is having a sponsor important in helping to ease depression? Does having a home group help overcome the isolation that so often goes with PTSD? Or is it simply sobriety—with or without Twelve Step involvement—that is the healing force?

Hopefully research in this area will continue to move forward, encouraged by the results we've examined here. In the interim, and based on these findings, it would seem appropriate to include parallel treatments for individuals who are dually diagnosed. A treatment plan for such an individual could include an intervention tailored to specific diagnoses such as depression or PTSD. It should also include a Twelve Step-based intervention aimed at facilitating and promoting engagement in a Twelve Step fellowship.

◆

Epilogue

This book has looked at what objective science has had to say about the effectiveness of the AA Twelve Step program of recovery, as well as the dynamic forces behind it such as sponsorship and spirituality. The bulk of this research is fairly new. Much of it was spurred by the findings of the U.S. Institute of Medicine's conclusion that AA, though ubiquitous, had not been the subject of rigorous research and its recommendation that such research be undertaken. That has been done.

The same group of prominent researchers from a variety of prestigious research centers who were cited earlier examined this emerging evidence on the effectiveness of AA and other abstinence-based mutual-help fellowships. Their review included AA, which remains the most prevalent fellowship that seeks to support recovery, as well as other fellowships such as Women for Sobriety, Narcotics Anonymous, and SMART Recovery that promote abstinence as their goal. Here is their summary statement:

> Because longitudinal studies associate self-help group involvement with reduced substance use, improved psychosocial functioning, and lessened health care costs, there are humane and practical reasons to develop self-help group supportive policies.

As we come to the end of this journey through the research on the Twelve Step model, what should we conclude? Is the AA model 100 percent effective—will it lead to recovery for every person, every time? Is it guaranteed to produce 100 percent sobriety?

The answer to that question, I'd suggest, is to be found not just in the AA Twelve Step model but in the way physical and mental illnesses as a whole are treated.

Thanks to the same kind of rigorous research used to evaluate the Twelve Step model, we know today that effective treatments for medical and mental illnesses are available. We have proven treatments for mental illnesses such as depression and PTSD. We have treatments for diabetes and heart conditions. But are these treatments effective 100 percent of the time? The truth it that these treatments all depend to a large extent on the willingness of the patient to follow through on them conscientiously. The best we can say, then, is that these treatments are likely to work if the individual works them.

It's also true that there are people for whom a Twelve Step program isn't compatible with their personality and lifestyle. However, as many of these people have found, if they can replicate the healing principles and practices in their lives that research has demonstrated makes these programs effective (such as honestly facing their addiction; finding support in family, friends, spiritual community, and so on—a power greater than self; dealing with unresolved emotional issues from their past; making restitution for harms done while using; and being of service to others), they too can find recovery. Conversely, if an individual opts not to comply with the requirements of treatment, does that mean the treatment doesn't work? Clearly not. As one example, consider diabetes. Although effective treatments for this disease have been available for a long time, a review by Alan Delamater, PhD, of the Department of Pediatrics at the University of Miami School of Medicine, points out that treatment non-adherence rates for chronic illnesses in general have long stood at roughly 50 percent, with those men and women diagnosed with diabetes even less likely to consistently follow regimens involving treatment that includes lifestyle change.

So it would appear from the research that the most appropriate answer to our initial question comes from the creators of the Twelve Step model: "Rarely have we seen a person fail who has *thoroughly* followed our path."

◆

References and Sources

Prologue

Institute of Medicine. 1989. *Prevention and Treatment of Alcohol Problems: Research Opportunities.* Washington, DC: National Academy Press.

Introduction

Joseph Nowinski, Ph.D. *"Frontloading" Among College Students: Motives and Outcomes,* Psychology Today blog, October 3, 2013, www.psychologytoday.com/blog/the-almost-effect/201310/frontloading-among-college-students-motives-and-outcomes-0.

A.A. Fact File. 1956. New York: Alcoholics Anonymous World Services (available at www.aa.org). Project MATCH Research Group. 1993. "Project MATCH: Rationale and Methods for a Multisite Clinical Trial Matching Patients to Alcoholism Treatment." *Alcoholism: Clinical and Experimental Research* 17:1130–45.

Project MATCH Research Group. 1996. "Matching Alcoholism Treatments to Client Heterogeneity: Project MATCH Posttreatment Drinking Outcomes." *Journal of Studies on Alcoholism* 58: 7–29.

Chapter 1

Alcoholics Anonymous. 2013–14. *The A.A. Service Manual.* New York: Alcoholics Anonymous World Services.

Alcoholics Anonymous. 2001. *Alcoholics Anonymous: The Story of How Many Thousands of Men and Women Have Recovered from Alcoholism.* 4th edition. New York: Alcoholics Anonymous World Services.

Alcoholics Anonymous. 1981. *Twelve Steps and Twelve Traditions.* New York: Alcoholics Anonymous World Services.

Alcoholics Anonymous. 2008. *Alcoholics Anonymous 2007 Membership Survey.* New York: Alcoholics Anonymous World Services (available at www.aa.org).

Alcoholics Anonymous. 2012. *Alcoholics Anonymous 2011 Membership Survey.* New York: Alcoholics Anonymous World Services (available at www.aa.org).

Alcoholics Anonymous. 1990. *Comments on A.A.'s Triennial Surveys.* New York: Alcoholics Anonymous World Services (available at www.aa.org).

Beckman, L. J. 1993. "Alcoholics Anonymous and Gender Issues." In *Research on Alcoholics Anonymous: Opportunities and Alternatives,* edited by B. S. McCrady and W. R. Miller. New Brunswick, NJ: Rutgers Center of Alcohol Studies.

Makela, Klaus. 1993. "Implications for Research of the Cultural Variability of Alcoholics Anonymous." In *Research on Alcoholics Anonymous: Opportunities and Alternatives,* edited by B. S. McCrady and W. R. Miller. New Brunswick, NJ: Rutgers Center of Alcohol Studies.

Alcoholics Anonymous. 2011. *The AA Member—Medications and Other Drugs.* New York: Alcoholics Anonymous World Services.

Chapter 2

American Psychiatric Association. 2013. *Diagnostic and Statistical Manual of Mental Disorders* (5th ed.). Washington, DC: American Psychiatric Association.

Moos, R. H., and B. S. Moos. 2005. "Paths of Entry into Alcoholics Anonymous: Consequences for Participation and Remission." *Alcoholism: Clinical and Experimental Research* 29 (10): 1858–68.

McKellar, J., E. Stewart, and K. Humphreys. 2003. "Alcoholics Anonymous Involvement and Positive Alcohol-Related Outcomes: Cause, Consequence, or Just a Correlate: A Prospective 2-Year Study of 2,319 Alcohol-Dependent Men." *Journal of Consulting and Clinical Psychology* 71 (2): 302–308.

University of Maryland–Baltimore County. 2000. *University of Rhode Island Change Assessment Scale: URICA.* Available at http://www.habitslab.edu/urica/.

Witbrodt, J., M. A. Yu Ye, J. Bond, F. Chi, C. Weisner, and J. Mertens. 2014. "Alcohol and Drug Treatment Involvement: 12-Step Attendance and Abstinence: 9-year Cross-Lagged-Analysis of Adults in an Integrated Health Plan." *Journal of Substance Abuse Treatment* 46, 412–19.

Kaskutas, L. A., L. Ammon, K. Delucchi, R. Room, J. Bond, and C. Weisner. 2005. "Alcoholics Anonymous Careers: Patterns of AA Involvement Five Years after Treatment Entry." *Alcoholism: Clinical and Experimental Research* 29 (11): 1983–90.

Timko, C., R. Billow, and A. DeBenedetti. 2006. "Determinants of 12-Step Group Affiliation and Moderators of the Affiliation-Abstinence Relationship." *Drug and Alcohol Dependence* 83, 111–21.

Timko, C., A. DeBenedetti, and R. Billow. 2006. "Intensive Referral to 12-Step Self-Help Groups and 6-Month Substance Use Disorder Outcomes." *Addiction* 101, 678–88.

Timko, C., and A. DeBenedetti. 2007. "A Randomized Controlled Trial of Intensive Referral to 12-Step Self-Help Groups: One-Year Outcomes." *Drug and Alcohol Dependence* 90, 270–79.

Majer, J. M., J. A. Leonard, A. M. Darrin, J. R. Droege, and J. R. Ferrari. 2013. "Categorical 12-Step Involvement and Continuous Abstinence at 2 Years." *Journal of Substance Abuse Treatment* 44, 46–51.

Buckingham, S. A., D. Frings, and I. P. Albery. 2013. "Group Membership and Social Identity in Addiction Recovery." *Psychology of Addictive Behaviors* 27 (4), 1132–40.

Erikson, E. 1965. *Identity: Youth and Crisis.* New York: W. W. Norton.

Haslam, Home, et. al. 2008. "Maintaining Group Memberships: Social Identity Continuity Predicts Well-Being after Stroke." *Neuropsychological Rehabilitation* 18, 671–91.

Chapter 3

Kaskutas, L. A., and E. Oberste. 2002. *MAAEZ: Making Alcoholics Anonymous Easier.* Berkeley, CA: Alcohol Research Group.

Kaskutas, L. A., M. S. Subbaraman, J. Witbrodt, and S. E. Zemore. 2009. "Electiveness of Making Alcoholics Anonymous Easier: A Group Format 12-Step Facilitation Approach." *Journal of Substance Abuse Treatment* 37, 228–39.

Subbaraman, M. S., and L. A. Kaskutas. 2012. "Social Support and Comfort in AA as Mediators of 'Making AA Easier' (MAAEZ), a 12-Step Facilitation Intervention." *Psychology of Addictive Behaviors* 26 (4), 759–65.

Nowinski, J. 2011. *The Twelve Step Facilitation Outpatient Program.* Center City, MN: Hazelden.

Nowinski, J., M. A. Baker, and K. Carroll. 1999. *Twelve Step Facilitation Therapy Manual: A Clinical Research Guide for Therapists Treating Individuals with Alcohol Abuse and Dependence.* National Institute on Alcohol Abuse and Alcoholism. NIH publication no. 94-3722.

Miller, W. R., A. Zweben, C. C. DiClemente, and R. G. Ryshtarik. 1999. *Motivational Enhancement Therapy Manual: A Clinical Research Guide for Therapists Treating Individuals with Alcohol Abuse and Dependence.* National Institute on Alcohol Abuse and Alcoholism. NIH publication no. 94-3723.

Kadden, R., K. Carroll, D. Donovan, N. Cooney, P. Monti, D. Abrams, M. Litt, and R. Hester. 2003. *Cognitive-Behavioral Coping Skills Therapy Manual: A Clinical Research Guide for Therapists Treating Individuals with Alcohol Abuse and Dependence.* National Institute on Alcohol Abuse and Alcoholism. NIH publication no. 94-3724.

Project MATCH Research Group. 1997. "Matching Alcoholism Treatments to Client Heterogeneity: Project MATCH Posttreatment Drinking Outcomes." *Journal of Studies on Alcohol and Drugs* 58 (1), 7–29.

Project MATCH Research Group. 1998. "Matching Alcoholism Treatments to Client Heterogeneity: Project MATCH Three-Year Drinking Outcomes." *Alcoholism: Clinical and Experimental Research* 22 (6): 1300–11.

Miller, W. R. 2005. "Are Alcoholism Treatments Effective? The Project MATCH Data: Response." *BMC Public Health* 5 (75).

Walitzer. K. S., K. H. Dermen, and C. Barrick. 2009. "Facilitating Involvement in Alcoholics Anonymous During Out-Patient Treatment: A Randomized Clinical Trial." *Addiction* 104 (3), 391–401.

Chapter 4

Alcoholics Anonymous (no date). "Comments on AA's Triennial Surveys." Unpublished document held by AA General Services Office, New York, NY.

Sanchez-Craig, M., D. A. Wilkinson, and R. Davila. 1995. "Empirically Based Guidelines for Moderate Drinking: 1-Year Results from Three Studies with Problem Drinkers." *American Journal of Public Health* 85 (6): 823–28.

National Institutes of Health. 2010. *Rethinking Drinking: Alcohol and Your Health.* NIH publication no. 13-3770.

Seitz, H. K., and P. Becker. *Alcohol Metabolism and Cancer Risk.* National Institute on Alcohol Abuse and Alcoholism. NIH publication available at http://pubs.niaaa.nih.gov/publications/arh301/38-47.htm.

Bagnardi, V., M. Blangiardo, C. La Vecchia, and G. Corrao. 2001. "Alcohol Consumption and the Risk of Cancer: A Meta-Analysis." *Alcohol Research and Health* 25 (4): 263–70.

Brooks, P. J., and S. Zakhari. 2013. "Moderate Alcohol Consumption and Breast Cancer in Women: From Epidemiology to Mechanisms and Interventions. *Alcoholism: Clinical and Experimental Research* 37 (1): 23–30.

Kishline, A. 1995. *Moderate Drinking: The Moderation Management Guide.* New York: Three Rivers Press.

Humphreys, K., and E. Klaw. 2001. "Can Targeting Nondependent Problem Drinkers and Providing Internet-Based Services Expand Access to Assistance for Alcohol Problems? A Study of the Moderation Management Self-Help/Mutual Aid Organization." *Journal of Studies on Alcohol* 62, 528–32.

Humphreys, K. 2003. "Alcohol and Drug Abuse: A Research-Based Analysis of the Moderation Management Controversy." *Psychiatric Services* 54 (5): 621–2.

Miller, W. R., and R. F. Munoz. 1982. *How to Control Your Drinking.* Albuquerque: University of New Mexico Press.

Miller, W. R., A. L. Leckman, H. D. Delaney, and M. Tinkcom. 1992. "Long-Term Follow-Up on Behavioral Self-Control Training." *Journal of Studies on Alcohol* 53, 249–61.

Bujarski, S., S. O. O'Malley, K. Lunny, and L. A. Ray. 2013. "The Effects of Drinking Goal on Treatment Outcome for Alcoholism." *Journal of Consulting and Clinical Psychology* 81 (1): 13–22.

Hall, S. M., B. E. Havassy, and D. S. Wasserman. 1990. "Commitment to Abstinence and Acute Stress in Relapse to Alcohol, Opiates, and Nicotine." *Journal of Consulting and Clinical Psychology* 58 (2): 175–81.

Magill, M., R. L. Stout, and T. R. Apodaca. 2013. "Therapist Focus on Ambivalence and Commitment: A Longitudinal Analysis of Motivational Interviewing Treatment Ingredients." *Psychology of Addictive Behaviors* 27 (3): 754–62.

Kelly, J. F., and M. C. Greene. 2013. "Where There's a Will There's a Way: A Longitudinal Investigation of the Interplay between Recovery Motivation and Self-Efficacy in Predicting Treatment Outcome." *Psychology of Addictive Behaviors.* DOI: 10.1037/a0034727.

Hamill, P. 1996. *A Drinking Life.* Boston: Little, Brown.

Knapp, C. 1996. *Drinking: A Love Story.* New York: Dial Press.

Alcoholics Anonymous. 2001. *Alcoholics Anonymous: The Story of How Many Thousands of Men and Women Have Recovered from Alcoholism.* 4th edition. New York: Alcoholics Anonymous World Services, 20, 108–109.

American Psychiatric Association. 2013. *Diagnostic and Statistical Manual of Mental Disorders* (5th ed.). Washington, DC: American Psychiatric Association.

Doyle, R., and J. Nowinski. 2012. *Almost Alcoholic: Is My (or My Loved One's) Drinking a Problem?* Center City, MN: Hazelden.

Holahan, C. J., K. K. Schutte, P. L. Brennan, C. K. Holahan, and R. H. Moos. 2014. "Episodic Heavy Drinking and 20-Year Total Mortality among Late-Life Moderate Drinkers." *Alcoholism: Clinical and Experimental Research* 38 (5): 1432–38.

Benton, S. A. 2010. *Understanding the High-Functioning Alcoholic: Breaking the Cycle and Finding Hope.* Lanham, MD: Rowman and Littlefield.

Chapter 5

Humphreys, K., S. Wing, D. McCarty, J. Chappel, L. Gallant, B. Haberle, T. Horvath, L. A. Kaskutas, T. Kird, D. Kivlahan, A. Laudet, B. S. McCrady, A. T. McClellan, J. Morgenstern, M. Townsend, and R. Weiss. 2004. "Self-Help Organizations for Alcohol and Drug Problems: Toward Evidence-Based Practice and Policy." *Journal of Substance Abuse Treatment* 26, 151–58.

Longabaugh, R., P. W. Wirtz, A. Zweben, and R. L. Stout. 1998. "Network Support for Drinking, Alcoholics Anonymous, and Long-Term Matching Effects." *Addiction* 93 (9): 1313–33.

Tonigan, J. S., G. J. Connors, and W. R. Miller. 1996. "Alcoholics Anonymous Involvement (AAI) Scale: Reliability and Norms." *Psychology of Addictive Behaviors* 10 (2): 75–80.

Miller, W. R., J. S. Tonigan, and R. Longabaugh. 1995. "The Drinker Inventory of Consequences (DrInC): An Instrument for Assessing Adverse Consequences of Alcohol Abuse." *NIAAA Project MATCH Monograph Series.* Volume 5. NIH publication no. 95-3911.

Wu, J., and K. Witkiewitz. 2008. "Network Support for Drinking: An Application of Multiple Groups Mixture Modeling to Examine Client-Treatment Matching." *Journal of Studies on Alcohol and Drugs* 69, 21–29.

Litt, M. D., R. M. Kadden, E. Kabela-Cormier, and N. Petry. 2007. "Changing Network Support for Drinking: Initial Findings from the Network Support Project." *Journal of Consulting and Clinical Psychology* 75 (4): 542–55.

Litt, M. D., R. M. Kadden, E. Kabela-Cormier, and N. M. Petry. 2009. "Changing Network Support for Drinking: Network Support Project 2-Year Follow-Up." *Journal of Consulting and Clinical Psychology* 77 (2): 229–42.

DiClemente, C. C., J. P. Carbonari, R. P. G. Montgomery, and S. O. Hughes. 1994. "The Alcohol Abstinence Self-Efficacy Scale." *Journal of Studies on Alcoholism* 55, 141–48.

Bond, J., L. A. Kaskutas, and C. Weisner. 2003. "The Persistent Influence of Social Networks and Alcoholics Anonymous on Abstinence." *Journal of Studies on Alcoholism* 64, 579–88.

Chapter 6

Alcoholics Anonymous. 2001. *Alcoholics Anonymous*. 4th edition. New York: Alcoholics Anonymous World Services, 59.

Kurtz, E. 1991. *Not-God: A History of Alcoholics Anonymous*. Center City, MN: Hazelden.

Alcoholics Anonymous. 2001. *Alcoholics Anonymous*. 4th edition. New York: Alcoholics Anonymous World Services, 62.

Alcoholics Anonymous. 1981. *Twelve Steps and Twelve Traditions*. New York: Alcoholics Anonymous World Services.

Galanter, M. 1999. "Research on Spirituality and Alcoholics Anonymous." *Alcoholism: Clinical and Experimental Research* 23 (4): 716–19.

Carroll, S. 1993. Spirituality and Purpose in Life in Alcoholism Recovery. *Journal of Studies on Alcoholism* 54, 297–301.

Mathew, R. J., V. G. Mathew, W. H. Wilson, and J. M. Georgi. 1995. "Measurement of Materialism and Spiritualism in Substance Abuse Research." *Journal of Studies on Alcoholism* 56, 470–75.

Mathew, R. J., J. Georgi, W. H. Wilson, and V. G. Mathew. 1995. "A Retrospective Study of the Concept of Spirituality as Understood by Recovering Alcoholics." *Journal of Substance Abuse Treatment* 13 (1): 67–73.

Miller, W. R., and J. C'de Baca. 2001. *Quantum Change: When Epiphanies and Sudden Insights Transform Ordinary Lives*. New York: Guilford Press.

Alcoholics Anonymous. 2001. *Alcoholics Anonymous*. 4th edition. New York: Alcoholics Anonymous World Services, 567.

Kelly, J. F., R. L. Stout, M. Magill, J. S. Tonigan, and M. E. Pagano. 2011. "Spirituality in Recovery: A Lagged Mediational Analysis of Alcoholics Anonymous' Principal Theoretical Mechanism of Behavior Change." *Alcoholism: Clinical and Experimental Research* 35 (3): 454–63.

Connors, G. J., J. S. Tonigan, and W. R. Miller. 1996. "A Measure of Religious Background and Behavior for Use in Behavior Change Research." *Psychology of Addictive Behaviors* 10 (2): 90–96.

Greenfield, B. L., and J. S. Tonigan. 2013. "The General Alcoholics Anonymous Tools of Recovery: The Adoption of 12-Step Practices and Beliefs." *Psychology of Addictive Behaviors* 27 (3): 553–61.

Montgomery, H. A., W. R. Miller, and J. S. Tonigan. 1995. "Does Alcoholics Anonymous Involvement Predict Treatment Outcome?" *Journal of Substance Abuse Treatment* 12 (4): 241–46.

Tonigan, J. S., and S. L. Rice. 2010. "Is It Beneficial to Have an Alcoholics Anonymous Sponsor?" *Psychology of Addictive Behaviors* 24 (3): 397–403.

Witbrodt, J., L. Kaskutas, J. Bond, and K. Delucchi. 2012. "Does Sponsorship Improve Outcomes above Alcoholics Anonymous Attendance? A Latent Class Growth Curve Analysis." *Addiction* 107, 301–11.

Chapter 7

Morgenstern, J., and M. E. Bates. 1999. "Effects of Executive Function Impairment on Change Processes and Substance Use Outcomes in 12-Step Treatment." *Journal of Studies on Alcoholism* 60, 846–55.

Beatty, W. W., R. Tivis, H. D. Stott, S. J. Nixon, and O. A. Parsons. 2000. "Neuropsychological Deficits in Sober Alcoholics: Influences of Chronicity and Recent Alcohol Consumption." *Alcoholism: Clinical and Experimental Research* 24 (2): 149–54.

Parsons, O. A., and S. J. Nixon. 1998. "Cognitive Functioning in Sober Social Drinkers: A Review of Research Since 1986." *Journal of Studies on Alcoholism* 59, 180–90.

Parsons, O. S. 1998. "Neurocognitive Deficits in Alcoholics and Social Drinkers: A Continuum?" *Alcoholism: Clinical and Experimental Research* 22 (4): 954–61.

Fein, G., and S. McGillivray. 2007. "Cognitive Performance in Long-Term Abstinent Elderly Alcoholics." *Alcoholism: Clinical and Experimental Research* 31 (11): 1788–99.

Chapter 8

American Psychiatric Association. 2013. *Diagnostic and Statistical Manual of Mental Disorders* (5th ed.). Washington, DC: American Psychiatric Association.

Petrakis, I. L., G. Gonzalez, R. Rosenheck, and J. H. Krystal. 2002. *Comorbidity of Alcoholism and Psychiatric Disorders.* National Institute on Alcohol Abuse and Alcoholism. Available at http://pubs.niaaa.nih .gov/publications/arh26-2/81-89.htm.

Fein, G. 2013. "Lifetime and Current Mood and Anxiety Disorders in Short-Term and Long-Term Abstinent Alcoholics." *Alcoholism: Clinical and Experimental Research* 37 (11): 1930–38.

Jordan, L. C., W. S. Davidson, S. E. Herman, and B. J. BootsMiller. 2002. "Involvement in 12-Step Programs among Persons with Dual Diagnoses." *Psychiatric Services* 53, 894–96.

Alcoholics Anonymous. 2011. *The AA Member—Medications and Other Drugs.* New York: Alcoholics Anonymous World Services.

National Association of State Alcohol and Drug Abuse Directors. 2001. *State Issue Brief No. 1: Current Alcohol Research in the Use of Medications as an Adjunct to Alcohol Treatment and Implications for State.*

Volpicelli, J. R., A. I. Alterman, M. Hayashida, and C. P. O'Brien. 1992. "Naltrexone in the Treatment of Alcohol Dependence." *Archives of General Psychiatry* 49 (11): 876–80.

O'Malley, S. S., A. J. Jaffe, G. Change, S. Rode, R. Schottenfeld, R. E. Meyer, and B. Rounsaville. 1996. "Six-Month Follow-Up of Naltrexone and Psychotherapy for Alcohol Dependence." *Archives of General Psychiatry* 53 (2): 217–24.

Weiss, R. D., J. S. Potter, D. A. Fiellin, M. Byrne, H. Connery, W. Dickinson, J. Gardin, M. L. Griffin, M. N. Gourevitch, D. L. Haller, A. L. Hasson, Z. Huang, P. Jacobs, A. S. Kosinski, R. Lindblad, E. F. McCance-Katz, S. E. Provost, J. Selzer, E. C. Somoza, S. C. Sonne, and W. Ling. 2011. "Adjunctive Counseling during Brief and Extended Buprenorphine-Naloxone Treatment for Prescription Opioid Dependence: A 2-Phase Randomized Controlled Trial." *Archives of General Psychiatry* 68 (12): 1238–46.

Bergman, B. G., M. C. Greene, B. B. Hoeppner, V. Slaymaker, and J. F. Kelly. 2014. "Psychiatric Comorbidity and 12-Step Participation: A Longitudinal Investigation of Treated Young Adults." *Alcoholism: Clinical and Experimental Research* 38 (2): 501–10.

Glassner-Edwards, S., S. R. Tate, J. R. McQuaid, K. Cummins, E. Granholm, and S. A. Brown. 2007. "Mechanisms of Action in Integrated Cognitive-Behavioral Treatment versus Twelve-Step Facilitation for Substance-Dependent Adults with Comorbid Major Depression." *Journal of Studies on Alcohol and Drugs* 68, 663–72.

Worley, M. J., S. R. Tate, and S. A. Brown. 2012. "Mediational Relations between 12-Step Attendance, Depression and Substance Abuse in Patients with Comorbid Substance Dependence and Major Depression." *Addiction* 107, 1974–83.

Kelly, J. F., R. L. Stout, M. Magill, J. S. Tonigan, and M. E. Pagano. 2010. "Mechanisms of Behavior Change in Alcoholics Anonymous: Does Alcoholics Anonymous Lead to Better Alcohol Use Outcomes by Reducing Depression Symptoms?" *Addiction,* 105, 626–36.

Trifﬂeman, E. 2000. "Gender Differences in a Controlled Pilot Study of Psychosocial Treatments in Substance Dependent Patients with Post-Traumatic Stress Disorder: Design Considerations and Outcomes." *Alcoholism Treatment Quarterly* 18 (3): 113–26.

Epilogue

Humphreys, K., S. Wing, D. McCarty, J. Chappel, L. Gallant, B. Haberle, T. Horvath, L. A. Kaskutas, T. Kird, D. Kivlahan, A. Laudet, B. S. McCrady, A. T. McClellan, J. Morgenstern, W. Townsend, and R. Weiss. 2004. "Self-Help Organizations for Alcohol and Drug Problems: Toward Evidence-Based Practice and Policy." *Journal of Substance Abuse Treatment* 26, 151–58.

Delamater, A. M. 2006. "Improving Patient Adherence." *Clinical Diabetes* 24 (2): 71–77.

Alcoholics Anonymous. 2001. *Alcoholics Anonymous.* 4th edition. New York: Alcoholics Anonymous World Services, 58.

Resources

Alcoholics Anonymous

Narcotics Anonymous

Twelve Steps and Twelve Traditions

Undrunk: A Skeptic's Guide to AA by A. J. Adams

Recovery Now: A Basic Text for Today (Anonymous)

Getting Started in AA by Hamilton B.

Finding a Home Group: A Guide to Choosing the Right Twelve Step Meeting for You by Jim G.

A Program for You: A Guide to the Big Book's Design for Living (Anonymous)

A Woman's Way through the Twelve Steps by Stephanie Covington

A Man's Way through the Twelve Steps by Dan Griffin

Sobriety: A Graphic Novel by Daniel Maurer, illustrated by Spencer Amundson

For Professionals

The Twelve Step Facilitation Handbook: A Systematic Approach to Recovery from Substance Dependence by Joseph Nowinski and Stuart Baker

Twelve Steps and Twelve Traditions

The Twelve Steps of Alcoholics Anonymous

1. We admitted we were powerless over alcohol—that our lives had become unmanageable.
2. Came to believe that a Power greater than ourselves could restore us to sanity.
3. Made a decision to turn our will and our lives over to the care of God *as we understood Him.*
4. Made a searching and fearless moral inventory of ourselves.
5. Admitted to God, to ourselves, and to another human being the exact nature of our wrongs.
6. Were entirely ready to have God remove all these defects of character.
7. Humbly asked Him to remove our shortcomings.
8. Made a list of all persons we had harmed, and became willing to make amends to them all.
9. Made direct amends to such people wherever possible, except when to do so would injure them or others.
10. Continued to take personal inventory and when we were wrong promptly admitted it.
11. Sought through prayer and meditation to improve our conscious contact with God *as we understood Him,* praying only for knowledge of His will for us and the power to carry that out.
12. Having had a spiritual awakening as the result of these steps, we tried to carry this message to alcoholics (others*), and to practice these principles in all our affairs.

The Twelve Traditions of Alcoholics Anonymous

1. Our common welfare should come first; personal recovery depends upon A.A. unity.
2. For our group purpose there is but one ultimate authority—a loving God as He may express Himself in our group conscience. Our leaders are but trusted servants; they do not govern.
3. The only requirement for A.A. membership is a desire to stop drinking.
4. Each group should be autonomous except in matters affecting other groups or A.A. as a whole.
5. Each group has but one primary purpose—to carry its message to the alcoholic who still suffers.
6. An A.A. group ought never endorse, finance, or lend the A.A. name to any related facility or outside enterprise, lest problems of money, property, and prestige divert us from our primary purpose.
7. Every A.A. group ought to be fully self-supporting, declining outside contributions.
8. Alcoholics Anonymous should remain forever nonprofessional, but our service centers may employ special workers.
9. A.A., as such, ought never be organized; but we may create service boards or committees directly responsible to those they serve.
10. Alcoholics Anonymous has no opinion on outside issues; hence the A.A. name ought never be drawn into public controversy.
11. Our public relations policy is based on attraction rather than promotion; we need always maintain personal anonymity at the level of press, radio, and films.
12. Anonymity is the spiritual foundation of all our traditions, ever reminding us to place principles before personalities.

The Twelve Steps of Alcoholics Anonymous are taken from *Alcoholics Anonymous, Fourth Edition*, 59–60. The Twelve Traditions of Alcoholics Anonymous are taken from *Twelve Steps and Twelve Traditions*, 129–87.

About the Author

Joseph Nowinski, PhD, is a clinical psychologist. He has held positions as assistant professor of psychiatry at the University of California–San Francisco and associate adjunct professor of psychology at the University of Connecticut. He is also a blogger for *The Huffington Post* and *Psychology Today*. Author of the *Twelve Step Facilitation Outpatient Program, Twelve Step Facilitation for the Dually Diagnosed Client,* and *The Family Recovery Program,* he also coauthored *Almost Alcoholic,* all books published by Hazelden. Nowinski has a private practice in Tolland, Connecticut.

About Hazelden Publishing

As part of the Hazelden Betty Ford Foundation, Hazelden Publishing offers both cutting-edge educational resources and inspirational books. Our print and digital works help guide individuals in treatment and recovery, and their loved ones. Professionals who work to prevent and treat addiction also turn to Hazelden Publishing for evidence-based curricula, digital content solutions, and videos for use in schools, treatment programs, correction programs, and electronic health records systems. We also offer training for implementation of our curricula.

Through published and digital works, Hazelden Publishing extends the reach of healing and hope to individuals, families, and communities affected by addiction and related issues.

For more information about Hazelden publications,
Please call **800-328-9000**
Or visit us online at **hazelden.org/bookstore**

Also of Interest

Recovery Now
A Basic Text for Today
In simple, practical language, this book combines current research with the timeless wisdom of Twelve Step program guides such as the "Big Book," *Alcoholics Anonymous*. Order no. 4265, ebook E4265

Now What?
An Insider's Guide to Addiction and Recovery
William Cope Moyers
A best-selling author and recovery expert answers the question "Now what?" for addicts and their loved ones as they share every step of the journey from contemplation through intervention, treatment, and recovery. Order no. 3982, ebook EB3982

Undrunk
A Skeptic's Guide to AA
A. J. Adams
With humor and revealing anecdotes, Adams introduces readers who "just don't get" Alcoholics Anonymous to the complete undrunk lifestyle, retracing his own often hilarious path toward transformation. Order no. 2944, ebook EB2944

The Addictive Personality
Understanding the Addictive Process and Compulsive Behavior
Craig Nakken
This classic, groundbreaking book brings depth to our understanding of how a person becomes an addict. Order no. 5221, ebook EB5221

For more information or to order these or other resources
from Hazelden Publishing, call **800-343-4499**
or visit **hazelden.org/bookstore.**